BACKROADS AND HIGHWAYS

MY JOURNEY TO DISCOVERY
ON MENTAL HEALTH

JOHN T. BRODERICK, JR.

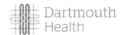

Copyright © 2022 by Dartmouth Health

Paperback ISBN: 9798218009540

Ebook ISBN: 9798218009557

All rights reserved.

No part of this book may be reproduced in any form or by any electronic or mechanical means, including information storage and retrieval systems, without written permission from the author, except for the use of brief quotations in a book review.

Cover photo by Mark Washburn

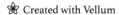 Created with Vellum

I dedicate this book to all the kids who warmly welcomed my message, to those brave kids who confided their stories and their pain, and to my family, especially my son, who inspired and supported my journey to discovery.

The net proceeds from the sale of the book will benefit the Broderick Fund to support psychiatric services at Dartmouth Health along with community education and advocacy efforts to overcome the stigma of mental illness.

FOREWORD

I found psychiatry when I was a medical student in the early 1980s and came to Dartmouth to train and to live in the beautiful Upper Valley region of Vermont and New Hampshire. I have been here ever since, working with colleagues to increase timely access to high-quality care for people who develop mental health or substance-use disorders. The illnesses we address are very common, very painful, often disabling and sometimes deadly. They are also very treatable: people get better with science-supported care. Yet, although psychiatric illnesses cause great suffering and touch all of our lives, action to make sure excellent care is there when we need it has been far from robust. In my class of 160 students at Harvard Medical School, only three of us went into psychiatry. Professional and family groups, who urge us to address this obvious problem, have often felt like they are lonely voices crying out in the wilderness.

How fortunate we are that John Broderick chose to speak! I met him at Dartmouth Health and have joined him at a few of his many, many public forums. His words struck me with force, and I could see that I was not alone. When he talks and writes, people lean forward to take in what he is saying. His story and his way with words touches our hearts. We realize we were suffering alone, but no longer have to. John uses simple language, humor and humility to describe his family's painful journey. As he lays out the facts and feelings, he opens the way for all of us to talk and connect. John Broderick invites us to leave the wilderness and come together. In his calm, kind voice, he notes that no one signs up for one of these illnesses. He invites us to join him in caring for ourselves and taking action to relieve the unneeded suffering all around us.

I am deeply honored that John asked me to write this forward to his wonderful book, which I urge you to read. Without fanfare or anger, he points out how far we are from the future that we desperately need—and that we can create. Discrimination against people who develop mental health and substance-use disorders is deeply baked into our society. It is present in our everyday language ("crazy people"), our moral attitudes ("it is all in your head") and in the structure of health care (mental health insurance carve-outs and payment rates that are much lower than the cost of providing care). John calls on us to address psychiatric illnesses with the same urgency and seriousness of purpose that we devote to cancer, Alzheimer's, and other illnesses that touch all of our lives. The process starts with changing how we see the world, but it does not end there. All of us—individuals, governments, health care organizations, insurers, and advocacy organizations—will need to take concerted action. As John says, the status quo is far from OK.

So, thank you, John, for this wonderful contribution to furthering a new national conversation about mental health. Whether we are students, educators, legislators, health care professionals, in pain or feeling well, young or old, we all benefit from your hard-won wisdom. We are so grateful for the important work you are doing—and that you continue to do.

> William C. Torrey, MD
> Raymond Sobel Professor of Psychiatry
> Interim Chair, Department of Psychiatry
> Dartmouth Geisel School of Medicine
> and Dartmouth Health

INTRODUCTION

For the last six years, I have been on a mission to begin a new, informed and nonjudgmental national conversation around mental health to finally, after generations of shame, stereotypes and stigma, change our culture that for too long and in too many ways has kept people and families suffering, ashamed and in the shadows. My travels have taken me to places I never would have visited, exposed me in very personal ways to a generation I have come to love, understand and admire, and opened my eyes and heart to the mental health challenges confronting today's youth. As a result of my often solitary, emotional journey on backroads and interstate highways, stopping at school gyms and auditoriums to engage students on mental health awareness, I have been profoundly changed. These students have opened up to me and allowed me in. They have shared their stories, their hugs and sometimes their tears. Their candor and emotional suffering have allowed me to find my real purpose in life. I am proud to be on their team and to advocate on their behalf. They are an incredible generation, but they are in need.

Once ignorant and complacent about mental illness and failing to see it in my own family, I have become impatient for real and meaningful change in the way we view and treat mental illness in America. We all need to be. Because I feel a very personal obligation to the thousands of students who were brave enough to share their struggles with me over these last many years and because meaningful change will require broad community support, I offer my chronicle of what I have seen and heard and felt on my journey to discovery. These kids are speaking to us, and we need to hear them. The status quo is neither their friend nor ours. We need to act. It's way past time.

Please note: All student and staff names used are pseudonyms; in some cases, I've also altered the location of schools so that they can't be identified. I have done both these things to protect privacy to the extent possible.

PREFACE

In my childhood, mental illness was never a topic for polite conversation. Certainly, I never heard it discussed. I was 10 when I learned that my best friend, who lived right across the street, had an uncle who was confined at the Danvers State Hospital north of Boston. Every adult I ever heard speak of that place—and every kid, including me—called it the "nut house." We must have thought that was funny. Nobody was ashamed to say that; nobody was embarrassed. Looking back all these years later, I realize that we all should have been ashamed. We all should have been embarrassed. But we weren't. I remember seeing the "nut house" only once as a kid from the passenger seat of my father's car as we drove past it one afternoon on a busy highway. Perched on a distant hill isolated and alone, it seemed a very scary place.

Often on Sundays in the summer, my friend's father would pick up his brother at the "nut house" and bring him to their house across the street. I dreaded the uncle's visits and never dared cross the street to play with my friend when he was there. I just didn't have the courage. From the safety of my front yard, I occasionally saw my friend's uncle looking at the flowers by the side of my friend's garage or just walking around their yard. He never looked at me, never spoke to me and never gestured to me. But as I watched from a distance, I was prepared to run inside my house at the slightest sign of danger. I was sure they kept people like him locked up to keep the rest of us safe. I have no idea why he was "imprisoned" at Danvers, but it likely was for something that would be treated today by outpatient psychiatric therapy. But back then, admission to a "nut house" had a very low bar. The way we treated suffering people like my friend's uncle was shameful. But I didn't know that then. We just separated them from the rest of us, locked them away and largely forgot them.

Everyone in my childhood town of 20,000 people had perfect mental health, or so I thought. Unless you were taken to Danvers, you were fine. Every marriage in my town was happy, too. Almost nobody got divorced. In my world, living under the same roof was the dividing line between happily married and unhappily married. If somebody was odd or different, it was somehow their choice. You did your best to avoid them. If anyone drank too much, they were an alcoholic—again, their choice. Veterans who returned home "different" were described as "shell shocked," which was not intended as a compliment. Anyone with a drug problem was an addict. They were seen as weak or flawed and different from the rest of us.

Given the stigma and shame associated with mental health challenges, it's no wonder people never talked about them or even acknowledged them. We must have all learned that when it came to mental health, it was better to conceal than to disclose. Besides, treatment was an illusion anyway —or so I thought. While there must have been mental health problems lurking behind many front doors in my middle-class town, those secrets never crossed the threshold. Family secrets were, after all, family secrets. The code of silence covered many problems. As I grew older, things changed some, but not dramatically. I never had anyone in my high school die by suicide, and no one at my college or law school did either. Mental health problems were still distant and largely out of view. Silence no doubt kept a lot of awkward moments at bay and also kept me in the dark.

I was so ignorant about mental illness that I never saw it when it crossed that road from my childhood decades later and took up residence in my own house. I was in my mid-30s, married and had two sons. Unbeknownst to my wife and me, our oldest son began experiencing symptoms of anxiety and depression when he was 13. We had no idea. He was a great kid who did well in school, played endlessly with friends in the neighborhood, and was blessed with incredible artistic talent. As it turned out, these many gifts helped him hide his illness for a long time. He thought what was making him feel different and often retreat to his room and his art was "just him" and that he would outgrow it. He didn't, and we never saw it until it was almost too late. His illness and our ignorance—coupled with our many mistakes, however well-intended—took my family on a journey I wouldn't wish on another living soul.[1] As much as we loved our son, we failed him. We should have seen more, done more and known more. We were, after all, the parents. We all paid a high price but thanks to my wife's incredible courage, my son's inner resolve, the grace of God and a lot of good people, we survived and have healed.

When unexpectedly given the opportunity to share my family's hard-earned knowledge about mental illness with others through the simple genius of psychologist Barbara

Van Dahlen's Five Signs campaign and the full support of Dartmouth Health, I embarked on the most important and meaningful work of my life. This book is about that odyssey of discovery—but, more importantly, it's about the thousands of brave young people I have been privileged to meet and hug in high school and middle school gyms and auditoriums all across New England. My journey has so opened my eyes and made me impatient to change not only the way we still view mental illness but also the shameful way we still treat it. With your help, much good can be done.

April 24, 2022

[1] See video at https://youtu.be/BHaYDn4cWzc, *Changing the Culture and the Way Mental Health is Viewed,* Dartmouth Health, August 21, 2020.

PART I

THE UNCHARTED ROAD AHEAD

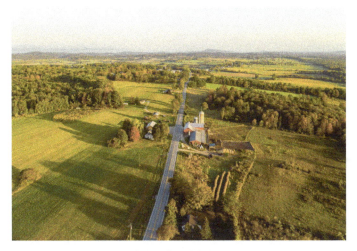

Photo credit: Caleb Kenna

One fall morning while I was driving to a mediation on the New Hampshire seacoast, my cell phone rang. It would be a call that would redirect my life. I had stepped down from my work at the law school at the University of New Hampshire several months earlier and begun my own mediation business. I had been a civil trial lawyer for 22 years and an appellate judge for 15 so I thought I must know something about settling cases. Besides, I liked trial lawyers and enjoyed being with them again. While I loved my time on the bench, I had missed the company of lawyers who had been a part of my everyday life for more than two decades. During my multiple-role legal career, I came to the view that it was always best to leave the stage before anyone asked rather than trying to hold the curtain open for one more act. So, in the late spring of 2015, I exited my law school position, stage right. Mediation seemed a perfect compromise. It was like leaving acting to work backstage. I would still be around the theatre but without the pressure of performing. I would also be able to slow down a bit. My wife, Patti, and I were looking forward to that.

When I took the call, I heard the billowing voice of Bill Gunn, a psychologist in charge of the department of behavioral health at Concord Hospital, from my dashboard. "John, Bill Gunn, how are you?" I had met Bill a year earlier during a private tour of his hospital in Concord. He had been unfailingly gracious and personable during my visit. Although his closely cropped white hair suggested that he was approaching his mid-60s, his boyishly handsome face and bright blue eyes made him appear years younger. Over the years, he had trained many medical school students from Dartmouth in family practice. I couldn't imagine why he was calling.

"I have a friend, Barbara," he told me, "who is a psychologist in Maryland with an office in Washington, D.C." As Bill told it, Barbara wanted to start a national mental health awareness campaign and had reached out to him to see if he would lead it in New Hampshire. "She wants New Hampshire to be the first state apparently, and she wants me to chair the effort here," he said.

"You're a perfect fit," I told him. "I am not surprised she asked you." As I was wondering why he was reaching out to share that news with me, he quickly got to the point.

"I told Barbara that I would help but that I didn't know enough people to chair it myself. That's why I'm calling. You know a lot more people than I do and your family's story was pretty public here. Are you willing to help me?"

"Help you?" I asked.

"Yes, as a co-chair," he said. "I know a lot of folks in the mental health community and after your 40 years in New Hampshire with your high-profile public service, my guess is that you'll know everyone else," he said with a chuckle.

My family's nightmare had begun 13 years earlier. It had almost destroyed us. I had only talked about it publicly twice. Once at a mental health conference at the Armory in Manchester several years earlier where Patti joined me for moral support and once at a gathering of New Hampshire lawyers. But I never really opened up at either venue. It was just too painful, and it wasn't just my story anyway. Not talking about it had proven the easier course and I knew that talking about it would only stoke my regrets and misgivings. Nobody ever asked and I never offered. Bill wasn't exactly asking, but a "yes" would make my silence much harder.

Without any time to reflect, I agreed to help. "I'm no expert but I do understand the journey of mental illness when it is not seen for what it is," I said. "At least I know what I didn't know and I realize the mistakes I made." I paused to gather my thoughts. "Maybe my ignorance could help other families see what I didn't and make better choices than I did."

"Why don't you let me know what works for you next week and we can sit down and talk about how to get this started," Bill replied with casual ease. "I've never done anything like this before but it would be fun to do it with you. I'll wait for your call. Safe travels to Portsmouth."

"Thanks, Bill," I said. "I'll get back to you with a date."

Then, as unceremoniously as he had arrived, Bill was gone. I was suddenly awash in the cluttered silence of hard memories that his call had unwittingly triggered. As I looked out at the passing fall landscape with its telltale splashes of red and yellow, I wasn't sure what I had just agreed to or even if I should have. Maybe, I thought, I should have waited to talk with Patti and my son. It had been their journey, too. Maybe they weren't ready. In fact, maybe I wasn't either.

It had been a long time since our family had begun its steep descent into hopelessness. After agonizing years of struggle, self-doubt, despair, self-blame and embarrassment, we had to claw our way back. We were weakened and vulnerable to be sure, but we had somehow survived. We were still a family. But I knew in my attempt to return to my everyday life that I had papered over some of the toughest and most devastating memories of those years; memories of endless days and nights when our lives were held prisoner to worry and regret. But despite my best efforts to outrun them, I couldn't. With the passage of time, some had mercifully lost their sharp relief, but they had never really disappeared. Some were seared into my brain, while others still woke me in the middle of the night. The guilt never left. It just burrowed deeper.

It's amazing what the mind does to help us heal but some pain never leaves; it has no outlet and no treatment. It imbeds itself and just lies in wait for the right trigger, the right moment. Even the comfort of happy family memories could be overtaken in an instant by the tragedy I didn't know then, but knew now, was coming. Bill's unexpected call had summoned those repressed memories and I found myself again forced to replay them, against my will, as I headed east to the ocean.

Maybe, I thought, the only way out of the pain and the grief that had weighed me down was to do the one thing I had tried mightily to avoid doing for more than a decade: talk about it. Silence and denial had brought no permanent healing. Maybe reaching out to face my guilt while sharing our family's cautionary tale to bring hope to others could turn my sadness into something positive.

When I got home that evening, I wasn't sure how Patti would react to Bill's invitation. I hesitated to bring it up. I was afraid it might open old wounds and incite flashbacks she kept to herself. She had been our family's strength from the very beginning. Patti had publicly endured the unimaginable during my post-operative days of induced sleep and was a constant companion at my hospital bedside in the weeks to follow. When she wasn't with me, it seemed she was in residence at the county jail trying to comfort our son and fighting for him to survive, too. She had been my day and night nurse at home during my months of healing and recovery and she was our son's companion whenever visits were allowed. Patti saw and did things I had been spared but, somehow, she kept everyone encouraged and moving forward. While I knew she cried alone many days on her way home from the jail and many nights lying awake after my pain medications allowed me to drift off, she never faltered; she never wavered. So, having me involved in a statewide campaign on mental illness that would undoubtedly bring our family's story back into the news with all the crushing memories it brought with it might be too painful for her to deal with. But she had earned the right to make that decision, and I would leave it to her.

After dinner, I asked Patti to go for a walk. The nights were getting cooler so we layered up. I was hoping the fall chill would clear my head and give me the courage to have what I knew would be a tough conversation. It would unearth memories we had tried to bury and force us to re-plow ground replete with failure and regret that had almost eviscerated us.

When we left the house that October night, I wasn't even sure I should have the conversation. Maybe it was best to leave well enough alone, as my mother might have said. My son, after all, had been out of prison for a decade. Although his life remained hard because of a felony conviction that followed him like an unrelenting enemy, bringing our story back up again might have no plus for any of us. But I knew that we had not fully healed. Maybe we had packed away our failures without confronting them. Maybe we needed to deal with them.

As Patti and I walked through familiar neighborhoods that evening with the sidewalks partially illuminated by the soothing light from walkway lamp posts and front porches, I was tormented by memories of years of incessant anguish. It was always alarming how close to the surface the darkness was. We had both felt incarcerated with our son and even when he walked free through the prison gates that September morning years earlier, a part of us remained behind bars. That place had changed us. I could still hear the cold echo of steel on steel. I remembered the sadness of visiting days and the painful realities they imposed on us.

As we were on our return leg home, I finally brought up Bill's call. I explained who Bill was and a little about the brief discussion I had with him that morning.

"What does he want you to do?" Patti asked cautiously.

"He told me that he wanted me to co-chair the campaign here. I suppose I will have to help raise money and reach out to others who could help us launch it," I replied with some uncertainty because I wasn't quite sure myself.

"Will our family's story be part of it? Will it be dredged up again?"

"I don't know for sure but if I get involved it likely will. I mean the only reason I would be doing the campaign at all is because of what we didn't know, the mistakes we made and the nightmare consequences we all suffered," I said, resigning myself to what I thought was going to be Patti's veto. "But it has been more than a decade since our family hit the front pages and we've never shared our side of the story," I said. "Christian is probably seen by a lot of people as a bad person and we know that's not true. Our own ignorance made things worse. He had an illness; he's not evil. Maybe the campaign could give us the chance to complete the picture."

Patti suddenly stopped walking. Her cheeks were light pink from the cold night air. Her blonde hair was peeking out from the edge of her wool hat that she had pulled down over her ears. I could see traces of her breath as she began speaking. She had endured so much since the assault. She was everyone's strength. But everyone has a breaking point. Maybe this would be hers. I could respect that.

"Maybe we should support it," she said to my surprise. "I

don't want other parents to endure what we did. I don't want other kids to suffer like our son did, either. Maybe the campaign will bring purpose to our suffering. Maybe our tale will be a wake-up call for other parents." Before I could respond, Patti resumed walking. "But we'll need to talk to Christian," she said. "Hopefully he'll understand why it could be important for others—and maybe it will help all of us heal, too."

The next morning, we spoke to Christian about it. "I don't need to be involved, do I?" he asked. "Don't get me wrong. I think it's a great idea. Nobody talked about mental health when I was growing up. There is so much people don't know or understand about mental illness. But I don't want to see my face in the papers again."

I assured him that he didn't need to do or say a thing and that I would protect his privacy if I was asked questions. "But I will learn more when I meet with Bill Gunn," I told him. "Look, when I know more, we can talk again. At this point, I really don't have any details about the campaign. If you decide as we learn more that you don't want me to be publicly involved, I won't," I told him.

"Thanks, Dad," he said. "But I just don't want to see my face in the papers again. The story makes me look terrible. It's hard enough getting any traction if you have a felony record. I can never forgive myself for what happened."

I met with Bill in Concord a few days later. Over lunch at a local restaurant, he told me about Barbara and his long professional friendship with her husband, Randy. They seemed like incredible people. Barbara's goal, according to Bill, was to make the five most common signs of mental illness as widely and commonly known as the signs of a heart attack or a stroke. Given my family's journey, fueled and exacerbated by my own ignorance, he didn't need to explain the importance of the nascent campaign. I suspected there were still a lot of parents like me and kids like my son who thought it was "just them."

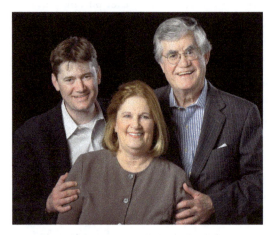

Christian, Patti, and John Broderick
(Photo credit: Paul Foley for The 99 Faces Project
99FacesProject.com created by Lynda Cutrell)

I just had no idea how many. Bill wasn't sure how the campaign would promote its message or even if it could find an audience. I wasn't either. But I committed to helping. I told Bill that although Christian was quite supportive of my involvement, he wanted to remain in the background. "He's been through a lot," I told Bill. "He doesn't want to see his face in print again." Bill fully understood. Before we parted, he said he would have Barbara call me. I still wasn't certain I was doing the right thing but there seemed no turning back now.

A few days later I was driving home in the late afternoon when Barbara called me on my cell. I pulled off on a residential side street so we could talk. By then I had learned what I could about her online. She was a highly respected psychologist in Washington, D.C., and was the founder of Give an Hour, a program for veterans and their family members afflicted with mental health challenges. Barbara had recruited a national network of psychologists and psychiatrists who agreed to donate hours of their professional time to treat this often overlooked and underserved population. Her efforts had been widely acclaimed and the Chairman of the Joint Chiefs of Staff Admiral Mike Mullen nominated her to be included on *Time* magazine's 2012 list of "The 100 Most Influential People." She was selected.

During our half-hour call, it was easy to see why. She was smart for sure but what impressed me most was her compassion for those suffering with mental illness and all those who loved them. I talked comfortably with her about my own son and what I had failed to see and understand. It was the first time I had ever done that. Somehow, it brought me a comfort that I wasn't expecting. She understood. Barbara had no clear plan on how to launch the Five Signs campaign in New Hampshire, but she did tell me there were some Five Sign posters in her daughter's Maryland school. Because I believed in the simple genius of her idea and felt my own stirring to do something to atone for my mistakes and the harm they caused, I committed to working with Bill to somehow move things forward. But when the call ended, I had no clear idea how to do that. I just knew that our lives would be changing again by whatever lay ahead. Almost unbelievably, the campaign had found me and despite my misgivings, I had enlisted. It all seemed so sudden. As I drove the remaining few miles home, I was nervous, yet inexplicably excited.

∾

OVER THE NEXT FEW WEEKS, Bill and I talked by phone several times about putting together a steering committee to help us create and lead the campaign. We shared names and connections. Some days, it all seemed too much. We had no money, no blueprint and no staff. Bill had a full-time job and less time to devote to planning and implementation than he wanted. But what we did have was a shared sense of the opportunity Barbara had given us and a quiet urgency to create meaningful change. I knew I could never have crafted the simple, straightforward, sidewalk-ready Five Signs message Barbara had, but as an old trial lawyer, I recognized its genius. It resonated with me. If we could assemble a statewide jury, I felt we could persuade them of its importance. Maybe change was possible. I knew we needed to try. It had all suddenly become quite personal. I felt I finally discovered a purpose for all my family's suffering. That alone was liberating.

Bill suggested I meet with Peter Evers, then-CEO of Riverbend Community Mental Health in Concord, to see if we could snag him to join our efforts. Peter was a transplant from England but had worked for years in Massachusetts in community mental health and, during his first few years in New Hampshire, had quickly risen as a respected public voice on all matters mental health. In short order, Peter and I got together at a local coffee shop on a cold, windy morning. Over muffins and hot chocolate, I sketched out a very tree-top outline of a campaign to deliver a statewide message about mental health. I was sure it sounded pretty abstract, but I knew Peter could help give it much-needed substance if he engaged. To my relief, he embraced it and offered to help. Peter held more cards that morning than he realized. If he had panned it, I might have wavered myself. He agreed to put pen to paper to begin outlining the campaign's content, and I agreed to begin the process of recruiting a steering committee and start raising money.

In the days that followed, I reached out by phone to the state's Commissioner of Health and Human Services, the state's Attorney General, the Commissioner of Corrections and countless others from public and private life. Every person I invited to join the committee agreed and strongly supported the broad mission I outlined for our work. Surprisingly, almost everyone I asked to join the campaign shared a mental health story about someone they knew or loved. That surprised me. The recruiting turned out to be far easier than I imagined. But I knew from my time as a law school dean that raising money for the campaign would be harder. I decided to begin by talking to hospital CEOs. Of all people, I thought, they should be interested. But I knew only one and not that well. So, I called the office of Dr. Jim Weinstein, president and CEO of what was then Dartmouth-Hitchcock—now Dartmouth Health—in the Upper Valley of New Hampshire to see if I could schedule a meeting. I was a bit nondescript about the purpose of the meeting but thought if I could see him and make the case, I could persuade others.

Jim and I met at his office several days later. He was in his early 60s with pure white hair, a warm and engaging smile and a radio voice. He made you feel instantly at ease. By background, Jim was an accomplished neurosurgeon, but I was confident his current duties kept him out of the operating room. I felt real pressure to get his help. I needed someone widely respected to invest in our campaign, and I wouldn't get a second chance. If Dr. Weinstein and Dartmouth Health were "in," I could leverage that endorsement throughout the New Hampshire hospital community. But if I failed here, it would likely give every hospital an out. We talked informally for about 20 minutes, and it was quickly obvious that Jim knew something of my family's story from a decade earlier. He was attentive as I shared my aspirations for the fledgling campaign. Jim told me he had colleagues across his career who had dealt with mental health challenges in their families, and he knew how stigmatized and embarrassed they often felt. He, too, believed we needed a new national conversation around mental health.

"How can we help?" he asked, as our scheduled time was drawing to a close. Knowing we wanted to raise $150,000, I asked if they could donate $25,000. I shared that Dartmouth Health would be the leader in the clubhouse if they were willing to commit.

"Let me see what we can do," he said, smiling widely. "I'll be back in touch." As I headed to the elevator, I knew that morning would be make-or-break, but I felt optimistic. Several days later, Jim called me. "We're in for $25,000, John," he told me with genuine pleasure in his voice. "Please keep us posted." After that, the rest of the money came easily from other New Hampshire hospitals. By the time we publicly launched the campaign in late May, we had exceeded our financial goal and had stakeholder hospitals, including the New Hampshire Hospital Association, vouching for our mission. Our campaign now had credibility. Little did I know that within a year of the launch, I would be working at Dartmouth Health as senior director of external affairs—and with their full support, I would be doing what I came to realize was the most important work of my life.

Once our fundraising goal was reached, where and how to launch our non-partisan, public awareness campaign was front and center. It had all happened faster than we thought possible. A member of the steering committee suggested we launch our public efforts at the New Hampshire State House. "Where in the State House would we do that?" I asked, thinking we might be able to get a hearing room off the main lobby. "I think we should ask the Speaker if we can use Representatives Hall," he said matter-of-factly. Representatives Hall is iconic in New Hampshire government and is the oldest legislative hall in America in continuous use. It is spacious, with high ceilings, rich colors and large, historic oil portraits adorning its walls. There are 400 theater-style tiered seats in that room and an ornate public balcony in its upper reaches. But I thought we would be setting ourselves up for defeat if we tried to fill a space that large on a workday—or on any day for that matter.

"Who will come to an announcement like this at 10 a.m. on a Monday?" I asked incredulously. "We might only get 20 or 30 people." Surprisingly, my pessimism wasn't shared. I was appointed to talk to the Speaker. Not only was he supportive of the idea, but he wanted to be there to welcome everyone. The Senate President did, too. We did what we could to get the word out through social media, radio interviews and a few articles in the state's newspapers, but it never had a stop-the-presses feel to it. On the big day, I was dreading walking into a near-empty hall. I hadn't slept much the night before worrying about turnout.

When Patti and I opened the rear doors to the chamber that morning, the room was packed. It was stunning and humbling. The launch exceeded all expectations. I was certain that Representatives Hall in all its subdued elegance had never hosted a more distinguished statewide gathering of leaders from so many disciplines. On a spring morning, our yet-to-be fully articulated awareness campaign had brought together our entire Congressional delegation, the House Speaker, the Senate President, the Governor, the faith community, our Supreme Court, the Attorney General, the President of the State Bar, the Commissioner of Education, hospital CEOs, doctors, nurses, mental health professionals, mayors, school superintendents, teachers, law enforcement, business community representatives and families. I couldn't imagine any other cause that would have drawn such a turnout on short notice. And the event that morning drew very favorable media coverage.

The successful launch made one thing abundantly clear: we had struck a nerve and unmasked a secret that had been hiding in plain sight for generations. As I looked out from the speaker's dais to welcome everyone, I saw clearly and starkly what I had failed to see for most of my life: mental health challenges impacted people and families almost everywhere and didn't play favorites.

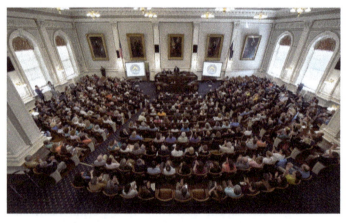

The mental health awareness campaign kicked off to a packed crowd on May 23, 2016, in New Hampshire's historic Representatives Hall at the State House in Concord. (Photo credit: Perry Smith)

It felt like a homecoming in Representatives Hall that morning where people were hugging, and laughing and sharing. There were also a few people crying. Patti was one of those. She had known the loneliness and heartache of our family's journey and because of her courage and my son's tenacity, we had made it through. She had nursed me back to health, encouraged my return to the court and ordinary life and held our family together. She had endured the unimaginable, so it was no surprise that she let her tears flow that emotional morning. But I was sure it was as consoling for her as it was for me to know that we had not been alone in that dreadful hopelessness all of those endless years. Many people and families were traveling with us on their own painful journeys. We just never saw them.

When Barbara Van Dahlen spoke that morning, she began by posing a question that immediately caught my attention. "If there is anyone in this chamber this morning," she asked, "who has never been touched by mental illness, either yourself, your family, your friends or your co-workers, please raise your hand." I had no idea what to expect. I reflexively scanned the room to get a rough count. In a matter of seconds, it was clear that no one was raising their hand. Apparently, every single person in that room had been touched by mental illness in some way because of someone they knew or loved. It seemed unbelievable to me, but not to Barbara. I asked her later how often she got that response. "It happens almost every time in almost every room where I ask the question, John. Just because people don't talk about mental illness doesn't mean people and families aren't dealing with it."

Barbara and her husband, Randy, came to the crowded reception with the Governor when the launch was over, and Barbara spoke passionately about the campaign and the need for change. I said a few words myself. It had been an amazing morning that held so much promise. After a small and memorable celebratory dinner that evening in Concord with the campaign leadership, I was up early the next morning to drive Barbara and Randy to the Manchester airport for their return flight to Washington. After we shared hugs and handshakes, they were off to their gate. As I walked through the terminal toward the parking lot, I was lost in thought. I knew that despite our exhilarating beginning, the real campaign would begin the next day and every day that followed. I had no idea if it could succeed or if it would matter. But I knew that if the launch proved anything, it taught me that there would be an audience for the campaign if we could reach them. We had to reach them. I was committed to trying.

Because Peter, Bill and I and the members of our steering committee had focused on trying to get people and the media to the campaign's launch, we never developed any clear plans for next steps.

We had hopes, but hopes weren't plans. We just didn't want the public announcement to be both the beginning and the end of the campaign, but we knew that was a possibility. We were in uncharted territory. Even if we had tried to reach a consensus on how the campaign should unfold, it might not have mattered. There were just too many unknowns. Above all, we hoped that our launch wouldn't fail and that somebody would reach back to help us find a path forward. There were no roadmaps or manuals to follow and no strategic plan to guide us. No other state had done what we were trying to do, so we couldn't learn through their experiences. Our approach was hopeful but pretty passive. But "opening day" brought a packed house and emboldened us to expect that others would embrace our mission, too. So, we waited hopefully. Thankfully, it didn't take long.

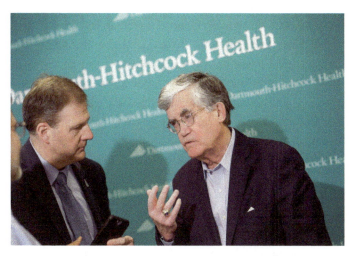

John discusses the state of adolescent mental health with New Hampshire Governor Chris Sununu. (Photo credit: Mark Washburn)

Our first contact came from NEA-NH, the state teachers union. In some ways, it wasn't surprising because the national and state data on youth mental health were disturbing. According to the results of the national Youth Risk Behavioral Survey (YRBS) from the Centers for Disease Control and Prevention (CDC)—a straight-forward, multiple-choice survey offered every two years to all public high schools since the 1990s—it was not uncommon to find that an alarming percentage of high school students were depressed, engaging in non-lethal self-harm and giving "serious consideration" to suicide. Similarly disturbing was the percentage of students who "had made plans in the last 12 months" to take their own lives. The rate of teen suicide was also increasing at an alarming rate. And none of the YRBS statistics included the unintended suicides from accidental drug overdoses and addiction. New Hampshire, for all its beauty and sense of community, had one of the highest per-capita death rates in America from opioids, the third-highest spike in teenage suicide in the country in recent years and a serious alcohol problem among adolescents. Schools were not the cause of the storm and were in fact doing their level best to combat it, but they were the everyday gathering place for all the kids who were swept into its destructive force. But we knew that getting into schools to speak to teachers and students wouldn't be easy —especially when the topic was mental health.

In the years to come and in ways I couldn't have imagined, the NEA-NH event opened doors that would lead me to meet and hug so many kids in so many schools who were suffering. The disturbing New Hampshire statistics I read about would, in time, have names, faces and dreams. But not yet having entered the thicket of young lives, I hadn't yet experienced the emotional impact of those encounters or how they would begin to reshape and refocus my life. The pained faces and confided journeys of the young people that would soon enough populate my life were largely invisible to me as I set out to challenge the shameful culture that had always surrounded mental illness. My hurtful ignorance and my own family's struggles were motivation enough at the beginning. But in the years to follow, the endearing trust and tears of those kids would come to sustain me on long solitary days of travel and talks. They would, in time, fuel my passion and growing impatience to challenge the injustice of mental illness that had gone unchecked for so many generations and had devalued the lives of so many people.

The NEA-NH invitation asked me to speak to a plenary session of teachers of all grade levels at a statewide workshop at a high school just outside of Concord. I arrived that morning not really knowing what to expect. I was told I had 45 minutes to speak. I had no idea how many teachers would be there. I had never really told my family's story before and just hoped I could. I had shared snippets but had never recounted the full journey. Almost 14 years had passed since that fateful Friday, and life all around us had moved on. But in many ways, my family's life had been stuck. I knew it would be hard to compress three decades and years of pain, fear and frustration into a manageable story that was both candid and inspiring. I also knew that I would need to be completely honest with myself and about my own shortcomings. There would be no place to hide in the retelling. There was a lot of blame to be shared, and I had to prepare myself to reveal my own mistakes. I wondered many nights whether I should be telling our story at all. Maybe, I thought, it would be best to just let more time pass and more memories fade. But mine wouldn't and my son's life would be frozen in a time capsule. The truth was far more nuanced and complex than incomplete newspaper accounts, and I wanted people to know about his courage, his decency and our family's healing. My son was smart and talented, but had been plagued by mental health problems that he never asked for and that had not been seen or understood for what they were until it was almost too late to change the narrative.

I felt an obligation to represent my son as the person he was and not just some one-dimensional figure who had injured his father and gone to prison. I knew who he was and wanted others to know that person, too. I owed him that. He deserved that. But I didn't want people to see me as whitewashing our family's tragedy or putting too fine a point on our story. I worked on my remarks for several weeks, sometimes as I was driving or lost in the isolating hum of my lawnmower or in the mindless distraction of washing my car. Memories would jump forward involuntarily looking for a place to be woven into my remarks. I wrote, rewrote and retold my family's story many times in my head before I began a bullet point outline on notecards. Patti and I talked many nights about what I should say before we turned out the lights on yet another day. It was a painful process for both of us, and it brought back memories we wanted to suppress. By now I could clearly see my mistakes and how they harmed my son. I was angry at my ignorance and inability to really see what was tormenting him—and us—and remorseful for the damage it caused. While I drew some solace from the cultural silence around mental illness for much of my life, and my good intentions, I couldn't exonerate myself. I had failed him and knew it. My son was paying the highest price of all of us and his otherwise promising life was shortchanged.

Christian knew about the campaign and was proud and supportive that I was so involved. He had shared many stories and observations about mental illness with me over the years since he left prison and what it felt like through his eyes when he thought it was "just him." Nobody had seen its intrusion but he began to experience its downward pull over time. His anchor, he told me, had been his art. He drew by the hour almost every day from a young age and, as he got older, often drew into the wee hours of the morning, sitting at his oversized desk in the loft above our garage when Patti and I were asleep. He enjoyed the stillness and focus art allowed him as well as the outlet it gave to his feelings. While drawing and creating, he didn't feel judged or in any way inadequate. Christian's art gave voice to who he really was. It brought him praise and admiration from others and permitted him to see himself in a positive light, if only for a while.

Over time, though, his mental illness created self-loathing. Some weeks were apparently worse than others.

He just couldn't do or be as he would have chosen and blamed himself. Sadly, his suffering was invisible to us because we weren't looking for the reasons behind his behavior but rather relied upon "common sense" explanations: creative people are different; he was up late because he needed to finish an art piece; he was likely tired or sometimes "just lazy." Years later he would say, "Dad, I wanted to be like everyone else, but I just couldn't. I thought I was too shy, too weak, too fragile and too deficient. I grew to hate myself because of it. I thought that was just who I was." Navigating school and college for all those years must have been overwhelming for him. What was merely uncomfortable or awkward for others was paralyzing and fear-filled for him. I was in awe of him because, despite his silent suffering, he earned both a bachelor's and a master's degree. I have no idea how he did that. Not knowing or understanding his obstacles is a guilt that will always remain with me.

    My mind was flooded with hopes and regrets as I pulled open the front door to Bow High School that morning. My stomach felt light. The lobby was teeming with teachers in casual clothes who were there for the daylong workshop. It seemed everyone was in conversation when I entered. I didn't see anyone I knew but it didn't take long for the president of NEA-NH to approach me. "Judge, honored to have you here today. The teachers are excited to hear your message." As we were shaking hands, he told me that he had come to the launch at the State House. "That was quite a crowd you drew, but this is an important topic. It needs all the discussion it can get," he said. As he was guiding me through the throng of teachers to the auditorium just off the lobby, a few of them thanked me for coming and a few others reached out to tell me they had come to the State

House. As we entered the still dimly lit auditorium, I wasn't sure whether I was speaking to everyone or just teachers who signed up to hear my talk. Before I had a chance to ask, he turned to tell me that I would be keynoting. "This place will be pretty full in about 10 minutes. There will be several hundred teachers here."

He showed me to my seat next to the podium in the well of the auditorium and then left me alone for several minutes as he was checking with his staff on logistics and sound. The auditorium was beginning to fill up, and there was a growing background noise generated by dozens of conversations happening simultaneously as teachers began taking their seats. The lights in that large room had been turned up and it was clear that a lot of teachers would be there. As I sat looking out at the gathering audience of strangers, I was struck by how vulnerable I felt and how unimaginable this moment was. I thought of my parents who had both died before our public nightmare began years earlier, and how surreal our journey had been since we lost them. They would never have believed today. I hoped they would have been proud of what I was doing. I thought of how strong Patti had been and how grateful I was that the Christian we loved had returned to us. I just hoped I had made the right decision to "go public." There was no turning back now. I could never have imagined my life would take me to this moment, but it had and I had chosen to be here. I had no idea what the reaction of the room might be to me or my talk. I wasn't even sure how I would feel when I was done.

After a gracious introduction, I stood and took my place behind the podium. The house lights had been lowered and much of the room was in silhouette. I placed my notecards under the podium's dim light, looked into the near-total darkness and began my talk. It had been such an unimaginable route to this morning. My family's star-crossed journey with unrecognized mental illness would have tested anyone's resolve but today, I thought, might be our way forward. Today might begin real healing for us and other families suffering more anonymously than we had. At least that was my hope. But I was far from certain. I didn't know most of the people in the audience; I knew it would be painful to share the intimate details of my family's struggles with them and expose my ignorance and mistakes to their judgments. "Good morning," is how I began. The room was pin-drop quiet. I was walking without a net; whatever happened, I was now on the wire.

"I am the last person in the world to be doing what brought me here today," I said. "But I see now what I didn't see or understand for most of my life. No one talked about mental illness in my childhood, in my neighborhood or in my town. Maybe that was your experience, too. I didn't really know anything about mental illness and didn't see it for what it was when it took up residence in my own house, in my own child. My ignorance about mental health harmed my own son."

After 35 minutes, I neared the end of my talk. The silhouettes staring back at me from the darkness hadn't moved, and I couldn't see the expressions on their faces. Fortunately, I hadn't stumbled, stopped or paused to compose myself as I feared I might. I was just relieved that I had made it through. As I was about to close, I realized that I hadn't really looked at my notecards after the first few minutes. I had wanted my remarks to seem as natural and unscripted as possible. I must have had faith that, left unchecked, my heart and conscience would join to tell the story. They had. But I was surprised at how drained I felt. Because I had never told our family's full story before, I had no clue whether or how it might connect with perfect strangers. As long as I was talking, I could delay the answer, but that comfort was short-lived. I ended by asking for everyone's help in changing the culture and conversation around mental illness. "If I could change it myself, I would, but I can't. But *we* could," I told them. "I hope I can count on your help. Together we can change and save lives. So many people are depending upon us. I know that now."

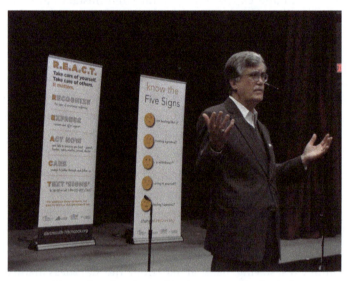

John speaks with students and faculty at Concord High School in Concord, NH, about the R.E.A.C.T. campaign for mental health. (Photo credit: Margaret Haskett)

As I was gathering my notecards, the house lights were turned up. I could now see the faces on those silhouettes who had sat patiently through my talk. Many were standing and soon everybody was standing and applauding. I felt both relieved and awkward. After all, I had just publicly recounted my family's horrific journey that was fueled by ignorance and mistakes—many of them mine—and the applause made me feel uncomfortable. I felt undeserving of their support, but in other ways I was grateful for it. They remained standing and applauding as I walked up the long side aisle into the lobby. I stayed for several minutes and spoke to many teachers as they filed out. Some opened up about their own stories in their own families while others just thanked me for sharing my family's journey. I received many hugs that morning and gave a few of my own. I felt free and inspired as I walked to my car. I couldn't wait to share my experience with Patti when I got home. She had, after all, made today possible in ways too many to count.

WITHIN THE MONTH, invitations to speak began to trickle in from a few high schools. The earliest asked me to speak to teachers and administrators, which I gratefully accepted. Because I had spoken to an auditorium filled with teachers at the NEA-NH weeks earlier, I felt confident that my talk would feel less uncomfortable in the retelling, at least before an audience of teachers.

After a few months, an invitation arrived from Pembroke Academy, a public high school just outside of Concord. The invitation, however, was different, asking me to speak to all 840 students. I was excited, but worried about whether young people would listen to me. I was, after all, the age of their grandparents, and I was unsure if they could relate to my story and my family's journey. It seemed a tall order to keep their attention for 40 minutes. I wasn't sure whether my message was right for a young audience or whether they would grasp my impatience for change. I had grown up in a different era with a strongly rooted culture of silence around mental illness. Maybe my perceptions were different than theirs. Maybe they wouldn't share my urgency or even understand it. But I accepted the invitation. I knew I would soon enough get answers.

When I arrived at the Academy that late fall morning, I had already decided to stick to the script. I couldn't devise a better way to tell our story and didn't want to soften its message or the history that set me on this path to try to change the culture and the conversation around mental illness. The principal was happy to meet me and proved a comforting host. After a few minutes of conversation in his office and brief introductions to the front office staff, he and I were off to check the sound system for my talk. "We couldn't get the whole school in our auditorium for your remarks today," he said. "It just won't hold everybody. So, we moved it to the gymnasium." To that point, I had never spoken in a gym. I knew it would be hard to do that effectively. I expected the sound system would be weak and the high ceilings would likely encourage my words to drift upwards to the rafters. Bleacher seats would not be comfortable, and I knew the kids would be easily distracted.

Nothing was lining up as I had expected. But I was there and had committed to speak, although I was now uncertain about it. As we entered the gym, the principal introduced me to a reporter from the *Concord Monitor*. My heart sank. I didn't need that added pressure. If my talk was not well-received that would be the story in the next day's paper.

The gym was cavernous. Nobody would have picked it as a venue for a serious talk, but it was the only option that morning. The school had set up a fixed podium with a goose-neck microphone on a small riser directly under one of the basketball nets. There were no folding chairs on the floor—only bleacher seats that stretched the full length of the gym on both sides. As the students filed in, we tested the mic. The principal seemed fine with it, but I had my doubts. Too late now, I thought. I was struck by how far away the kids were once they took their seats. From all my years as a trial lawyer, I knew how important eye contact was to the art of persuasion, to making a real connection with people. That was clearly not going to be possible in this room.

As I took my place behind the podium after the principal's kind introduction, I realized I had never spoken to an audience the age of these students in a place less conducive to making a connection. I felt deflated but was grateful for the silence that ensued once I began talking. I could at least hear my voice; whether the students could, I wasn't sure. Near the end of my talk, I was struck by how attentive they had been but had no idea what that meant. Maybe they were straining to hear me or perhaps they were uncertain why I was sharing my story with them at all. As I concluded, I asked for their help to change the culture and erase the stigma around mental illness. I assured them if they joined me, they could change things and save the lives of a friend, a classmate, a family member and, someday, maybe one of their own children. I told them their voices really mattered.

When I stopped speaking the room was motionless. It looked like a painting. The principal, standing just behind me at the edge of the gym floor, stepped up on the riser. Silence. I felt so exposed and uncomfortable as he shook my hand. Obviously, I thought, my remarks had fallen flat. Maybe the campaign would end here. But after several endless seconds of deafening quiet, the students began to stand on both sides of that gym, now smiling, applauding and whistling. It shocked me—and it shocked the principal, too. The applause continued for a full minute with the sounds echoing off the block walls. They had heard me, they understood and they agreed with me. I was inspired by them and grateful beyond measure for their support. As their applause died down, I realized they had shown me the way forward for the campaign: I had to reach students. They would help me force the culture change. They were ready. I was ready now, too.

SEVERAL WEEKS later in response to another invitation to speak to students at an even larger high school in central New Hampshire, my Pembroke experience was replayed. On that morning, I stood in the center of the gym floor with bleachers almost touching the ceiling on both sides. The room was bigger and the ceiling was higher than Pembroke. I talked for 40 minutes, moving slowly, turning gradually trying to keep everyone's attention on both sides of that gym while adjusting my mic to make certain students could hear me. They listened intently.

When I concluded, they spontaneously stood and applauded. Teachers were standing, too. I knew they weren't applauding me. But they were clearly as impatient for change as I was. That's what their applause was telling me. Mental health issues affected so many students in so many schools and very often someone in their families or circle of friends. It was familiar to them. They knew as I knew that silence and shame had helped no one for generations. These kids were smarter and braver than I was at their age. I was proud they were embracing the message and knew they would lead the change we needed. On mornings like that, I wished I were younger to be part of the movement I was fully confident they would create and drive.

Once my talk ended, several students began to walk toward me at center court as others followed classmates to the gym's exit and their next classes. That morning would be the first time students approached me after my remarks. A few thanked me for coming, a few gave me high fives while a dozen or more wanted to confide. It was very humbling to experience their openness because I was a stranger to them, but based on my honesty in presenting my story, they trusted I would listen without judgment.

The first student I spoke to that day had long hair, a baseball cap on backward and the height and build of a linebacker. He was several inches taller than I was and many muscular pounds heavier. I immediately noticed that his eyes were moist. He looked lost. Without introduction, he asked, "Can I give you a hug?" His request startled me.

"You're a lot bigger than I am," I replied with a smile, trying to process his offer. "Hug away." He squeezed me like a life preserver in heavy seas. Over the next two minutes, he shared his own mental health journey with me. I could barely believe he was in school. When he finished, his head now inches from mine and his eyes tearing, I said to him, "You may be the toughest guy I have ever met. Will you let me return the hug?"

"I'd love that," he quickly replied. As I was hugging a linebacker I had just met and trying to lessen his pain, I realized for the first time that the road ahead would not be easy. But I knew it would be important.

Over the next six years, I would travel almost 100,000 miles by car in northern New England in all types of weather. I would speak more than 690 times, with more than 300 of those talks in middle schools and high schools where I spoke to more than 86,000 students, grades six through 12. Every place I went, the kids listened and responded. After every talk, I would stay to speak to students who lined up to share with me. Sometimes I would still be in the gym or auditorium an hour after my talk ended. The students often had wet eyes and cracking voices but they wanted to share with someone who would not blame or dismiss them. I would often hug them to support their bravery or ease their suffering, and many times they reached out to hug me first. Their trust and candor emboldened my impatience for change. After all of those encounters, I wished I had known more about mental health when my oldest son's suffering, silent and unseen, was disrupting and wantonly changing his young life. He deserved so much better. I should have known more. I should have understood. I was, after all, the parent.

In the years that followed my talk at Pembroke Academy, I never visited a school to talk to students where I wasn't deeply touched and affected by what I heard and by the hugs I shared. But some moments, stories, and faces stayed with me and remain with me to this day. I feel an obligation to share them.

IT WAS STILL DARK when I got up one morning and the house had the chill of late October. Tepid sunlight first appeared as I set out on my drive north to a mid-size high school in Meredith, a beautiful town on the shores of Lake Winnipesaukee in central New Hampshire.

The lake's foliage was past peak that day, and its tapestry was soothing as I descended the long, steep lakeside hill populated with shops, restaurants and rental offices into the center of town. Meredith's shoreline was dotted with million-dollar homes, boathouses, private docks and a handful of restaurants. The less wealthy lived on the town's backroads further inland. On most weekends in October,

Meredith was swelled by tourists in search of the best local overlooks to enjoy the breathtaking kaleidoscope of a New Hampshire fall. The few elegant hotels around the cove with their prized outdoor balconies were always at full capacity. The winters there had their own rhythm, too, albeit quieter; once the sheltered bay froze over, "bob houses" for ice fishing popped up, and everyone looked forward to the New England Pond Hockey Classic that drew big crowds in late January. On winter's windy days, the colorful sails of iceboats—raised by brave souls dashing across the lake—added a much-welcomed flair to the white and gray of winter. Occasionally, you would even hear the muffled sound of a small plane landing on the ice if conditions were right. Without question, Meredith was quintessential small town New England.

The principal of the high school there had heard my talk a few months earlier at a statewide administrators' conference and followed up. The campaign had progressed organically. People would hear my talk and reach out or someone who had heard me would recommend me to a colleague. Sometimes there would be a story in the newspaper that generated interest. However fortuitously it was catching on, I had promised myself I would accept every invitation, however inconvenient, to keep the momentum going. I now had speaking opportunities lined up into March. Our mental health awareness campaign was slowly but surely finding a path forward.

As I turned onto the entrance road for the high school shortly before 8:00 a.m., I spotted a large, glass-enclosed sign with black magnetic letters that read, "Welcome Chief Justice Broderick." A very nice touch, I thought, but whenever you are greeted by something as thoughtful as that, it adds a bit of pressure. I hoped that when I was driving away in two hours, I would feel deserving of that special greeting. Every school had differences, to be sure. Some were small and rural and some regional; some were wealthy, while others were struggling with very tight budgets. I had even spoken at a few private high schools with sticker-shock tuitions. But I was happy to visit all of them. I found my reserved parking space, grabbed my Five Signs rack cards and posters and headed to the front entrance of the school.

Although I didn't know it then, my visit here would foreshadow dozens and dozens of school visits in the months ahead where kids were facing gremlins and the counselors and administrators were discouraged. I would come to learn that schools were trying to help too many kids with too few resources, too few referral options, too few counselors and too little support from parents and school boards. Budgets never stretched far enough to deal with mental health.

When I told the principal that day that high schools seemed to be different than when I attended in the 1960s, he chuckled. "If you haven't been in a high school in the last ten years, you've never been in a high school," he said matter-of-factly. This wisdom would be affirmed at every school I visited. The change began at the front door: kids had codes to enter and guests didn't. At every school, I would have to buzz my way in after explaining who I was and why I was there. Almost all the schools had cameras to size you up before you heard the telltale click of the lock sliding aside. The clicking sound always jolted me, reminding me of the sound made by the steel door into the inmate visiting room. I would be asked to sign in at a window usually just inside the entrance door and be issued a badge or a clip-on identification card of some kind.

At one rural high school in far northern New Hampshire —where you might think no one ever gave a thought to security—I had to pose for a picture to add to my badge. That was a first. Once I was finally cleared to enter the front lobby of most high schools, it was common for me to see a uniformed and armed police officer sometimes casually talking with students, sometimes just surveilling the surroundings. That shocked me the first few times I encountered them, but I understood why the police were there. The Columbine High School shootings in Colorado two decades earlier and the many senseless school shootings since then made police officers as visible in our schools as custodians. While this would have been unimaginable in my childhood schools, it was now commonplace. They even had new names: instead of police officers, they were called "school resource officers."

I reflected on how much had changed since I was their age. Anyone could have walked into my town's high school without a question being asked. All I needed to do was remember my locker combination, and I never saw a police officer in the halls. No student would have those memories now. On a visit to another high school a few weeks earlier, I had to walk past a marked police cruiser parked 20 feet from the front door facing out to the parking lot. I knew it was there to discourage violence, but that fact alone was unnerving. It couldn't help but affect kids. In my childhood, we practiced getting under our desks to protect ourselves from a surprise attack by the Soviet Union. But I knew they were a long way away and that our military would make sure they wouldn't get to us. We never had to practice "active shooter" drills for a circumstance where somebody would come into our school with a gun and try to kill us. The only drills I remember were fire drills. Most often they were a welcome relief from the classroom. These kids had worries I couldn't have imagined. They had to be affected by them. They would have affected me.

After greeting the office staff, the principal and I headed down a maze of corridors to the auditorium. At every school I visited, I was struck by how clean they were. The floor tiles were always glistening. At least that part of high school hadn't changed. On this day, for some reason, the polished floors evoked childhood memories of accompanying my father on winter Saturday mornings to the high school in our town where he was assistant principal. We always had the huge building to ourselves, and it was an adventure for me to roam the hallways and stairwells even unlocked classrooms while my father caught up on work.

"Don't touch anything on a teacher's desk" was my only admonition. My father spent most of his adult life teaching before moving to administration to make a little more money to help put my sister and me through college. I knew he liked teaching more but he made the move for us. That's who my father was. I always felt close to him on mornings like this. I thought how ironic it was that after years as a trial lawyer and judge at the end of my professional career I would be spending much of my time in high schools just as he had. Even more ironic was that I would consider my work talking to students about mental health the most important work I had ever done. My father, a gifted teacher, no doubt felt the same when he walked away from teaching that last day. All of my current work had been so unplanned and unexpected. But in an odd yet comforting way, it made me feel close to my father.

As we were entering the auditorium, the principal turned to me and said, "We think some eighth-grade students will be joining us this morning. Their buses should be arriving in a few minutes." I was pleased to hear that some middle schoolers would be there for my talk. I hadn't spoken at any middle schools yet and wondered whether my message would connect with them. Today would be one small baby step in that direction.

As I sat watching the kids file in and take their seats, I was thinking that when I was their age, nobody like me had ever spoken at my high school. Truth be told, nobody like me would have ever been allowed to speak. Mental health was just not on anybody's radar. In my childhood, you were either in a "nut house" and unseen, or you were fine and part of everyday life. So mental health challenges didn't exist didn't exist—or so I thought. Maybe kids today would see me as out of touch. I hadn't raised children for decades. While still lost in thought reflecting on where I was and why I had come, I suddenly realized that the principal had almost finished introducing me. I stood up to face the students. They were warmly applauding. There were even a few loud whistles. Standing in front of them, I had flashbacks to my own high school. But I thought I looked older than they did when I was their age. They just seemed so young to me. As they grew older, I knew the retelling of their high school years would be distilled down to a handful of friends they cared about, a few teachers who made a difference, a small number of successes, a few disappointments and a few really important moments. I just hoped that somebody here this morning might remember some judge who spoke in their school all those years back and told them that it was OK not to be OK, that help was possible that could change their lives and that they certainly weren't alone.

The auditorium was full, but with the lights dimmed the faces darkened and turned to outlines after the first 10 rows. But I could at least make eye contact with a few students.

That helped me tell my family's story in a more intimate way and allow me to read their reactions. This morning, as was true every time I spoke to kids, I wondered how many of them would relate to what I was about to say and how many were dealing with mental health challenges at that very moment. I was certain there were more kids there from single-parent homes than was true among my high school classmates and more kids being raised by grandparents than in my hometown years earlier. There were likely more kids who had experimented with drugs and who may have known or lost someone who had been caught up in New Hampshire's growing opioid problem—maybe somebody in their own family. The kids all looked homogeneous but behind the smiles and warm welcome, I knew there were differences. As I began my remarks, I confessed my near life-long ignorance about mental illness and asked for their help in changing the culture of shame that has surrounded it. You could almost feel the students lock in. They could relate. When I finished, they stood and applauded, this time with more commitment than when I began. They knew.

I stayed 45 minutes after my remarks to be with the students who came forward to talk. I never picked a time to stop. I always stayed until the gym or auditorium was empty. I knew I had to be present for those brave kids. They had listened to me, and I felt an obligation to listen to them however long it took. As hard as it was for me to recount my family's story and my own failings as a parent in front of perfect strangers less than a third my age, the stories the kids shared were always harder for me to deal with than my own. They had many years ahead of them, and I wanted to change their trajectory in some small way to alter their outcome—to lessen their fears. I wanted them to know that I believed them, that their pain was not their fault and that help was possible. I wanted them to know they should accept no shame or blame for something they had not chosen. They had a health problem; nothing more.

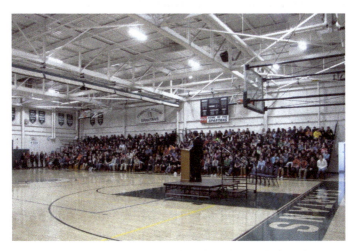

Students pack the gymnasium to hear John's talk at Pembroke High School in Pembroke, NH. (Photo credit: Margaret Haskett)

I had told so many kids, "I could have your problem. I didn't do anything special not to have it, and you didn't do anything to deserve it." I always listened intensely to the kids who confided in me. They could sense that I cared about them, however briefly we talked. That was important to me. That's why I came. We bonded at some level in those candid moments. I was humbled by their courage and their trust. I blocked out everything around me and ignored my own emotional exhaustion to hear them—to really hear them. These kids who didn't know me before I arrived that morning were now sharing their personal pain, often within earshot of their classmates. They were so anxious to share. Sometimes they would approach me with a friend who they said was with them for moral support. Sometimes their friend could have used moral support, too. But they came. Somehow, they all found the strength to open their lives to let me in. They would begin our encounter by hugging me or thanking me for coming to their school and talking about "it" or for "sticking up for kids like them." They often had wet eyes.

Some were barely able to speak. I had never experienced anything remotely close to the confessor status they were bestowing on me unceremoniously but so personally. While I couldn't change their lives in those fleeting moments, I could, I thought, at least validate their openness and encourage them to reach out and talk with someone they trusted.

On days like this, I regretted that I hadn't been present and aware of my own son like I was for these kids. I only wished he could have named his challenges and talked to me about them. But I probably should have known more and seen more. I was plagued with doubt, too. Maybe I would have discouraged his confessions and just told him life could be hard or that being a teenager was not easy for anyone and that he would grow out of it. Maybe I would not have been as enlightened or compassionate as I was now. After a day spent hugging kids, the course of my family's life, so impacted by my well-intended mistakes and my son's unnamed and then misnamed treatable illness hung on me like dead weight. At least these kids were talking about it even if much of the adult world around them was still afraid, disbelieving or uninformed. These kids would change the shameful culture around mental illness as they grew into adulthood. I was sure of that. But I wanted the pace of change to quicken. I wanted fewer casualties and fewer battle scars. I was weary of reading about teenage suicide, of embracing kids in real time who had tried to kill themselves and of seeing the fear and suffering of kids who should have been embracing the fleeting wonder of life at a young age.

Feeling depleted but grateful that my visit had done what I hoped, I found myself alone, gathering my materials from the stage that was waist-high behind me. Everybody had gone on to class. Even the principal was missing. I must have really overstayed my welcome, I thought. But it had been worth it. The auditorium was in almost total darkness as I headed toward the illuminated exit sign above the room's side door. After a few steps, I heard a soft voice.

"Judge Broderick, can I talk with you?" At first, I couldn't see where it was coming from. Then I saw a young girl standing up in the darkness. She was in the middle of the front row. I walked toward her.

"Sure," I said, "but aren't you supposed to be in class?"

"No," she replied. "They said I could stay to talk with you if you have time."

"Of course, I do," I said supportively. "Why don't we just talk here?" I sat down next to her leaving an empty seat between us. "What's your name?" I asked her.

"Rebecca," she said, "and I am 13."

To put her at ease, I told her that I was once her age and that I had wanted to stay as young as she was for my whole life. "How's that working out for me?" I asked. She grinned.

"I'm in the eighth grade," she said proudly.

"Did you hear my talk this morning?" I asked.

"Yes," she said nervously, "I heard all of it. I think I have some mental health problems myself. That's what I wanted to talk about."

"What are they?" I asked softly as I leaned gently forward to better see her face.

"I feel very anxious and very depressed," she said. "I just don't like the way I'm feeling."

"That's not easy, I know," I said to reassure her, "but at least you are aware of what your problems are. My son didn't understand he had mental health problems. He thought it was just him. And I never saw his problems either. So, you are better off than we were, and that's good." She was intensely studying my face as I spoke. "Have you spoken to anyone about how you're feeling?" I asked. "That would be a good thing to do."

Casting her eyes abruptly to the floor, she said quickly, "I spoke to my dad about it." Then she paused. I was waiting for more but she remained silent.

"That's good," I said. "What did he say?"

Her eyes remained down. "He told me he didn't believe in mental illness and that I should just get over it," she said, sounding forlorn.

I had heard that refrain from other kids in other schools on other days. "Don't be too hard on your dad," I said trying to lift her spirits. "I am sure he loves you very much. But he grew up at a different time. I was probably like your dad once myself but I understand more now."

She was studying me. "Can I ask you something that is really bothering me?" she said with some urgency.

"Of course," I replied. At this point, I felt I had known this young girl for a long time. She was so courageous.

"Am I the only kid in this school that is suffering like I am? Am I the only one?" she asked. She was deadly serious.

I smiled to calm her. "No," I said. "I know statistically you're not. Twenty percent of all the kids you go to school with have some type of mental health issue, and even more know or love somebody who does. The important thing is that you get help. Help really matters. You don't need to feel as badly as you do." She looked at me appreciatively and seemed genuinely relieved.

"Thank you for telling me that. I thought I must be the only one," she replied.

"Do you have a teacher or a counselor in your middle school that you like?" I asked.

"Yes. There is a teacher I really like that I feel like I could talk to."

"Great," I said. "Are you willing to tell her what you have shared with me? Even if she can't help directly, she will get you to the right person. Maybe she could even reach out to your dad, too, and help to explain things to him."

She hesitated for a second. I hoped I hadn't lost her. "I will," she finally said. "I will."

"Will you promise me you will see her today?" I asked.

"I will see her before I leave school today. I promise." She began to stand, then hesitated briefly. "What will I say to the teacher when I see her?" At that moment, she revealed that she was still a child even though that had been easy to forget over the last few minutes of painfully honest conversation worthy of any adult.

"This is what you should say," I began. "Tell her a judge spoke at the high school this morning and that he ordered you to come see her and that you think he had the power to do that." Now she was smiling widely, revealing her braces.

"Can I really say that?" she asked.

"That's exactly what you should say," I told her. "I'm counting on you."

With that, she stood up, paused awkwardly to hug me, and began walking up the center aisle. "Thank you for talking to me," she said. Then she disappeared into the darkened auditorium.

She made every mile I had traveled that day worthwhile.

I hoped she found the help she needed. I hoped today was as important for her as it was for me.

I HAD BEEN GIVING my talk for more than a year by the time I received my first invitation to speak at a middle school. It came out of the blue in a call from a New Hampshire principal. He had apparently talked to a friend who had heard me speak at a community forum across the state.

After briefly introducing himself, he got right to the point. "I was told by a close friend that I should get you to speak to my students," he said. "My friend heard your talk. He thought it would be really important for my students and staff to hear you. Can we get a date for you to do that?" he asked. "I would be happy to pay something. I just don't know what you charge."

"The good news is that I don't charge anything," I told him, explaining that I now worked for Dartmouth Health, "and they make it all possible. So, there is no cost to you."

He quickly followed up. "If you could come, it would be terrific. I would like to make a small gift, though," he said, "if that's OK."

"That would be very much appreciated," I replied, "but don't feel obligated."

"What you're doing is important," he said. "I am happy to make my small contribution. Have you ever spoken at a middle school before?" Just the way he said it made me wonder if I should just politely decline.

"Not yet," I told him, "but I have spoken at a lot of high schools. So, I have to defer to you on whether you think your students might be interested in hearing from me. You'd be a far better judge than I am." I was half hoping he would reconsider. He didn't.

"I think the kids should hear your talk. My friend was impressed. We see mental health issues at our school," he said. "A lot of kids these days are suffering." I was surprised by that—they were in middle school, after all. In time I wouldn't be surprised at all, but at that moment, it caught my attention. We talked for a few more minutes about what I had been seeing and experiencing during my high school visits, and before we hung up, I had accepted his offer to speak. But honestly, I wasn't sure I should have. I was plagued with reservations.

High schools were one thing but talking to middle school kids seemed like uncharted territory. I wasn't even sure I could give the same talk to kids as young as the sixth grade that I had been giving to adults and high schoolers, but I also knew that I didn't want to water down my remarks. I wondered if parents of middle schoolers would push back when their kids shared my story when they got home. I dreaded the prospect of blank stares and disinterested gazes from young kids pressed together on uncomfortable wooden bleachers in an early morning assembly. How would I feel if they just sat there with quizzical expressions when I finished? As I feared it, I knew I had to expect as much. I was far from certain that I was ready for the acid test of trying to hold the attention of young kids. After all, I would likely be the oldest person who had ever spoken to them at their school.

My family's story was hard enough to tell as it was but it would be painful, almost disrespectful I thought, to share it with kids who I feared might look bored or perplexed. As a trial lawyer, I had grown comfortable speaking to juries—but they were older and had taken an oath to at least listen before deciding. Speaking to a jury of middle schoolers with a million more immediate things on their mind and still years away from even being eligible for a driver's license was intimidating. If I spoke and it went badly, maybe word would spread and my invitations would begin to dry up. But I had committed to come so I just steeled myself and hoped for the best. After a lot of thought, I decided that I would not change my remarks for the younger audience. I would give the same talk and live with whatever happened.

A few days before I was scheduled to speak, I got a message on my voicemail from the principal. My first thought was that he had reconsidered his invitation or that parents or teachers were concerned that it might be too much for the kids to handle. I returned his call quickly, half-expecting bad news. "I just wanted to confirm you'll be here on Thursday," he said in a very upbeat tone.

"I will be there. I am looking forward to it," I said in a way to convince both of us. Truth be told, I had been having second thoughts about it for weeks but I knew I had to do it. It was too late to back out.

"We are excited you're coming. I just wanted to let you know that I invited a small middle school nearby to join us on Thursday. They're about 15 miles away. They will be busing them over. Maybe I should have asked you first but I thought the more students the better. I hope that was OK," he said.

"That's fine," I replied. "I'll see you Thursday." Increasing the size of the audience should have pleased me, but instead it just intensified my worries.

After a restless night, I drove 90 minutes that Thursday morning on winding country roads to the middle school in western New Hampshire. I was surprised by how uncomfortable I felt. I wasn't nervous exactly because I had given my talk dozens of times by then, but today I wasn't sure that my message would resonate. I just had no sense of the audience I would soon be opening my life to. I was so invested in the campaign, I didn't want to risk derailing it by reaching out to middle schoolers who might not even understand what I was saying or why I was saying it. On the ride that morning I experimented out loud with ways to soften my remarks to avoid shocking or upsetting anyone while hoping to save myself from the unpleasantness I was afraid was coming. But I was unsure what, if any, changes would work. I finally gave up trying to put myself in the kids' shoes. I was flying blind, and I knew it.

The principal greeted me warmly in his outer office, graciously introduced me to his assistant and then guided me into the corridor for our short trip to the gym. "I think the kids will enjoy your talk this morning," he said warmly. "The teachers have told them about you and why you are visiting our school. They have never had anyone like you come to speak with them." He mentioned that he wasn't expecting any behavior problems from the kids but that the teachers would keep a close watch just in case. As we entered the gym with the kids filing in around us, he said, "I hope the handheld mic will be okay. The sound isn't always great but it should work." My worst fears were being realized: a young audience that could misbehave and a sound system that could have problems. When the kids took their seats, the principal walked to the middle of the gym floor to quiet them. Once he had their attention, he told them how proud the school was to have me there and asked them to listen to what I had to say. I then walked out from my bleacher seat to take the mic. "Good luck," he whispered, as he made the handoff and walked toward the bleachers. I knew I would need it.

I knew the first minute or two would be the toughest. If I could get their attention, I thought I could hold it. But the sixth graders, sitting slightly apart in their own section, looked so young to me. At that moment, I was thinking, in turn, how old I must look to them. What delighted me was that the kids seemed engaged once I began speaking. I walked forward to be closer to them. If I had stayed in the middle of the gym floor, I thought I would lose them. I wanted it to seem like we were having a conversation even though I would be the only one speaking. Luckily, it seemed to work. I didn't see anyone fooling with their neighbor or sharing hushed comments with a classmate. I spoke for my 40 minutes as I always did. They paid close attention, and for that, I was more grateful to them than they could ever have imagined.

When I finished my remarks with my usual plea for their help, they began clapping. It grew in intensity, reverberating off the gym walls. They had not only listened—they had understood and agreed. They had been the scariest jury I had ever spoken to but no longer.

I stood by the exit as they filed out. Some students thanked me for coming and some even shared how much it meant to them personally. One little boy told me that my talk was "awesome." One seventh-grade girl hugged me on her way past. "Thanks," she said. Several kids looked like they wanted to stop to talk but classes were resuming and the buses would soon be arriving to take the visiting kids back to their school. But my visit had been a success. These kids understood what I never would have understood at their age. As reassuring as that was, it was also concerning. Their lives were more challenging than mine had been.

After saying goodbye to the principal who seemed pleased with how things had gone, I walked to my car in the parking lot not far from the front entrance. As I did, I saw dozens of kids scattered in small groups across the striped macadam. At first, I was confused as to why they were outside, but I quickly remembered that they were the visiting middle schoolers waiting for their buses. I sat in my car for a few minutes checking my e-mails. I was answering one when I was startled by a rap on my driver's side window. My first thought was that I must have parked in someone's reserved spot. When I looked up, I saw a boy whose face was inches away from my window. Maybe I was blocking the bus, I thought. I lowered my window to talk.

"Judge," he said with an infectious smile, "I loved your talk. I love what you're doing." It startled me. And it embarrassed me, too. I had been concerned these kids might not even relate to my story.

"Thanks," I shot back. "You guys were great." He had made my day. I carefully backed up and as I cleared the cars on either side, I saw 10 or 12 of his classmates. As I drove slowly past them, they began applauding. "Thank you," they were yelling, "thank you!" At the end of the first row of cars, I turned left toward the parking lot's exit. Almost in front of me was a larger group of kids. They began applauding, too. I could hear their thank-you shouts through my closed windows. I smiled and waved to them, and they continued to applaud until I reached the exit. I had never experienced anything like it. They taught me more than I taught them that day. Because of the incredible gift they gave me that morning, I would make many middle school visits in the months and years to come.

∼

NEW HAMPSHIRE IS KNOWN MOSTLY for its foliage, its "Live Free or Die" state motto and its incredibly beautiful mountains and lakes. But it is also home to a few of the very best private high schools in America. They are not immediately visible to the casual observer nor necessarily in the spots you might imagine. Some are in or near the mountains or up narrow backroads off two-lane rural highways: some nestle close to the downtown of small historic villages where it's sometimes hard to distinguish the downtown from the campus and some are on the outskirts of larger communities. But wherever you find them, they all share the common view that they are academically stronger, more whole-student focused, more engaged in the larger world and better feeders to elite colleges than virtually all public high schools. And they are almost always right about that. But, because most of their students don't go home every day, these schools expect more independence and resilience from kids than schools where students walk or take the bus. Sometimes kids are able to rise to that challenge, but sometimes, through no fault of their own, they aren't.

Being a product of public education in a middle-class town and knowing almost no one who went away at the end of the eighth grade to an elite high school, I never had the occasion to visit prep school campuses before the awareness campaign brought me to those environs. Invitations from schools of privilege were slow to come but in time they arrived. The delay was not unexpected. Mental health had never been a topic of discussion in the everyday America where I grew up—never mind in the world of privilege and outsized expectations that was private prep schools. There, especially, mental illness needed to be hidden. A clean record for the ride to the top was important. But it sometimes came at a high price.

I remember my first visit to a private high school. The opportunity came unexpectedly from one of the school's deans, who was extending the invite on behalf of all the students. She had apparently read of my efforts to start a new conversation around mental illness and suggested my name to a group of students who were organizing a full-day, no regular classes, campus-wide event. The school had encouraged these in-depth discussion days for several years so that students could select topics of larger importance—like race, sexual identity and climate change, among others—to explore the choices and challenges they presented. In their own idealistic way, these "thought" days were a call to action. But whatever topic was selected, it was the students who chose it. Nothing like that ever happened in my high school, where we pretty much did what we were told and followed time-worn schedules with few options. So, I was impressed. But what astounded me was that the students had chosen mental health awareness for their day of learning and reflection. Maybe things really were beginning to change, I thought—at least among young people.

"We'd like you to keynote their day," the dean told me. "You would be addressing the entire school that morning in the auditorium. Several faculty will be there," she said. "They want to hear your talk, too." I was delighted and immediately accepted.

When I arrived on campus several weeks later on a sun-splashed morning, I did my best to follow the map I had found online. Finding the right entrance was my first challenge but then making the right road choices quickly followed. Reading maps had never been a strength of mine so I was delighted to find parking lot C after just a few minutes of uncertainty. The dean had arranged for me to have breakfast with eight students before my talk and was planning to join us, as well. I had no idea why these students were chosen but assumed they had organized the day.

As I walked hurriedly across campus for my meeting, I was struck by how lush it seemed. The mostly brick buildings were sited in groves of trees and thick shrubbery amidst winding walkways. Shade was generously dispersed over the freshly mowed lawns. It felt like I was visiting an elegant small town. I remember thinking as I walked along that I wished my parents had been wealthier or that I had been smarter—or both—after viewing the extraordinary world around me. I had to stop a few unsuspecting headset-wearing students for directions but I found my building. Fortunately, two students were there to meet me just outside the front entrance. "Judge Broderick, we are so delighted you can join us this morning," one of them said. They warmly shook my hand. They had no idea how happy I was to have found them after my uncertain odyssey across the sprawling campus.

"Thanks for inviting me. I just hope I don't disappoint," I said as we walked into the building. We followed a meandering route to our private breakfast spot that had large windows overlooking the manicured grounds. The dean and a half dozen other kids were there to greet us. They all made me feel very welcome. We gathered our buffet breakfasts and reassembled around a large oak table. The dean spoke first to welcome me and to give me some history on these thought days. I then asked the students to introduce themselves and tell me about their interests and plans. Each student spoke briefly. They were just as articulate as I thought they would be. They were bright, personable and had come from across the country to study here. Many national figures had attended this school, too. Maybe one or more of these students would join that exclusive club in the years ahead. They were all impressive.

As our current events chatter wound down and before we all left for the auditorium, I asked two of the kids closest to me where they wanted to go to college. One said Yale and the other, a junior from the Midwest, told me quite directly, "My mother wants me to go to Berkeley." I was tempted to reply that I hadn't asked where her mother wanted her to go but I didn't. I just wished her luck. She seemed like a wonderful kid but it was disturbing that she didn't really hear my question. When I was her age, I aspired to a specific college, too, but that aspiration was mine—supported by my parents to be sure, but ultimately my choice. But I was sitting at a table of high expectations and substantial achievement and, as I came to realize over time from my awareness campaign visits to other very privileged places, they often came with very different pressures than I ever experienced growing up.

I walked over to the auditorium in the company of a senior boy from our breakfast group. He was from New York, he told me. The sun was warming as we headed across campus. He had been one of the leaders behind this day. I asked him how it came about. "Mental health is a concern for a lot of my classmates but we don't talk about it much. There's still a lot of stigma," he said with resignation. "So, we thought we could use this year's day away from classes to learn more about it and get people talking. That's why we wanted you to come," he said. As we walked, he opened up about himself. "I lost my mother to suicide last year," he told me.

"Oh my God," I said, "I'm so sorry to hear that." I hadn't been prepared for that disclosure. "I'm sure your mother was a wonderful person and very proud of you," I told him.

But I knew my response was weaker than he needed—and weaker than I wanted.

"She was both of those," he said, "but she was depressed. I miss her every day." He told me she had died over the winter break months earlier. "When I came back to school everyone had heard something about it but nobody wanted to talk about it. It was almost like nothing happened and here I was in pain, and I remained quiet about it."

"I'm sure people didn't know what to say so they just avoided it," I suggested, "but I'm sure they felt uncomfortable because they knew you were suffering. Many people still don't understand why someone would take their own life. I understand now because I have a much better knowledge of depression and what it can unleash. I hope you are talking to a counselor," I told him. "You have been through so much." He didn't respond.

As we entered the balconied auditorium, he said his father was visiting and would be there for my talk. I stood with the young man in the well of the auditorium just below the stage as the seats on its floor and overhanging balcony filled. When he introduced me to his classmates, he told them briefly of my career as a judge and as Chief Justice in New Hampshire but he made it clear that my visit was only to talk about mental health awareness, what I had learned from my mistakes and what I now saw. I realized anew that morning that my former title opened doors to what had become the most important work of my life; without that part of my resume, I knew I might not be there at all.

I used a handheld mic and made my usual presentation, which held their attention. They stood and applauded. Even here, I thought. After I handed the mic back to my young host, he waited for quiet to resume. Without preamble, explanation or context, he then posed a question to the entire school. "If there is anyone here this morning who has a mental health problem or someone you love has a mental health problem, would you please stand up?" Those were the only two categories: you or someone you loved. No place to hide there. No ambiguity. I had no idea what to expect. I had never heard that question asked by a student of his classmates at any school I had visited. But here, where the Ivies were well within reach for many of these kids, I wasn't convinced many would stand. It just seemed like a disclosure no student would want to make so publicly and so personally before their classmates, especially in front of faculty. I watched intently to see if anyone moved.

After a brief stillness, kids began standing. First in groups of two or three and then in larger numbers. Within 15 to 20 seconds, those standing began to outnumber those who were seated. And the standing continued. By the time it stopped, almost all the kids were on their feet. It looked like no more than two dozen remained in their chairs. Maybe they were too afraid, I thought, or too proud or just honest. But the visual was stunning.

"Thanks for being so honest," the senior graciously told his classmates. "I think it is important that everyone realizes that mental health challenges affect so many of us and the people we love." He then asked everyone to be seated. "We want to conclude this morning's program by asking several students to talk about their own mental health challenges," he said. At first, I thought I had misheard him. "I intend to lead off," he said, as he ascended the stairs to the stage and walked to the podium. He reached down briefly to grab his notecards on the shelf below.

"I lost my mother to suicide last year," he began, "and when I returned to school, nobody talked about it, and I didn't talk about it either." You could have heard a pin drop.

I was awed by his courage. He was candid about how their silence had pained him and how tough his recovery had been. After two minutes he yielded the podium to another student and then another until eight had spoken about how they were navigating their own mental health challenges. It was the breakfast group I had met with just two hours earlier. That's why they were chosen to host me. I understood that now. Although I barely knew them, I was so proud of each of them for what they were risking, admitting and managing in their own lives. Mental health challenges were hiding in plain sight even here, and because of some brave and smart students that morning, everyone was forced to see it and begin the process of reassessing old stereotypes.

After talking with several students who wanted to thank me for coming and huddling with my breakfast group, where I told them how courageous I thought they were, I gathered my few materials to head out. But for one person, I had the auditorium to myself. The gentleman was about my height but maybe 15 years younger. He walked toward me with a friendly grin. "That was terrific," he said with enthusiasm, "thanks for sharing all that with the students." As we shook hands, he introduced himself as the head of the school's counseling office. He had been there for a while and when I asked about his background, he told me he was a physician. Of course, I thought, private schools like this could afford a doctor. We chatted about mental health for several minutes and about what he was seeing on campus.

He was quite impressive. As we spoke, I wished every school could have someone like him. When we reached the front steps, I stopped to ask him a question.

"Doctor," I said, "what's it like if you need to reach out to a parent here because you have concerns about their child's mental health?"

He paused ever so slightly as if to make certain he ordered his thoughts. "Some are fine and supportive," he said, "but most aren't as receptive as I would hope."

"What do you mean?" I asked.

"Usually, the first question they ask is, 'have you written anything down, have you told anyone about this?'" It was clear what they were worried about.

"Not what you need," I said, reflecting back on what he had shared.

"Not at all," he replied crisply. "Not at all."

We shook hands goodbye and I descended the steps to cut across campus in search of my car. The grounds still looked as beautiful as they had when I had arrived but, in some ways, they looked less idyllic and less perfect to me now. I couldn't get the image of all those kids standing out of my head, and I couldn't forget the breakfast kids and their amazing courage.

Fortunately, I found parking lot C. As I was driving through the campus gates, I knew we were failing people with mental health challenges everywhere—and not just in poor schools or bad neighborhoods or broken families. We were failing them here. Even here.

ALTHOUGH RELATIVELY FEW IN NUMBER, my visits to private schools were ones I particularly looked forward to. Since I never reached out to them to solicit an invitation—nor any school for that matter—I was always a bit surprised when a prep school requested that I come to campus. I had no network for access to private schools and so was always interested in the back story of how and why they reached out when an invitation arrived. Despite my interest, I rarely found out. Nonetheles, though I looked forward to these visits, I still held my breath: I didn't know whether my message for their accomplished students, a message the school administration had not personally seen nor heard, would be consonant with school ethos and expectations. The coin of the realm in these select schools was their success in developing the full potential and inner gifts of their students. Watching some of those students hug a stranger and open up about personal suffering after listening to a talk on mental illness might prove to be an unsettling image to the administration. But it was a risk I was certainly willing to take.

Public schools had differences to be sure but for a casual visitor like me, they often looked and felt the same. Private schools had certain commonalities, too, but they often had richly different histories and stories. You had the sense that many were competing for the same students and although cordial toward each other, they were living in more of a zero-sum world than public high schools ever did. Because of that jockeying, I respected private schools that took the leap of faith to invite me.

I received an invitation late one spring to speak at a very well-respected prep school in a neighboring state. It was in a rural setting but conveniently close to the interstate. I knew of its reputation and even had a few law partners who had children who attended, but there had never been an occasion for me to be on campus. When I arrived that warm late April day, my first assignment was to find the dining hall for a pre-talk lunch with the head counselor, a woman named Beth, and a few faculty members. Arriving just a few minutes before noon, I had little time to spare but fortuitously my task turned out to be easy. I just followed the dozens of students crisscrossing the broad campus with its many white clapboard New England-style buildings heading toward a low, sleek modern structure of brick and granite. I figured that must be the Commons where lunch was served. I grabbed the first available parking space and hurriedly followed the groups of students heading that way.

I met Beth just inside the Commons front entrance. "Delighted you could come, Judge," she said. "I think everyone is looking forward to it." But time was short so she quickly ushered me toward the buffet lunch line crowded with students. "We need to be in the auditorium in about 30 minutes, so we will have to eat light," she said with a chuckle. "I hope you're not too hungry." Fortunately, I rarely ate before I spoke so no lunch would have been fine with me but it would have felt impolite to share that since lunch had been part of her invitation.

As we inched forward with one eye on the clock, I was struck by my lunch choices posted in colored script on top of the glass shelving displaying a wide array of hot and cold foods and multiple salads. It would be hard not to find something you liked here, I thought. There was even someone behind the counter willing to throw something on the grill if you wanted. The lunch offerings seemed more fit for a restaurant than any school cafeteria I was familiar with. Not exactly the plastic trays and "eat it or go hungry" menu of my high school years. Even my college, where several nights a week we were served "mystery meat," couldn't pretend to compare with this spread.

As I stood waiting with the students, I couldn't help but notice that they were gazing down toward the dim light and solitude of their iPhones. I wondered how many appreciated the exceptional surroundings they lived in here or even viewed them that way. I also wondered how many of these kids might be intimidated by them. Some of these kids no doubt were here on need-based scholarships so this had to be a different world for them. But with a price tag north of $65,000 a year to be enrolled here, everyone in line had to know that much was expected of them.

I never had that added pressure when I was their age attending a public high school. I wasn't sure how I would have handled it, but I knew I would have felt more pressure. When my turn came, I grabbed a salad and a small plastic container of dressing and followed my host into the much noisier main dining area where we joined a few teachers who were almost done eating. We tried to talk over the background noise but after a few minutes, we broke camp to head out across the quad to the auditorium. My salad went largely untouched.

As Beth and I bounded down the Commons steps, she spotted someone she knew and hollered out his name. He waved and she beckoned him over. Turns out he was the headmaster. She introduced us briefly and he welcomed me to the campus. "Judge," he said, "I have to check on something in my office quickly but I am coming to your talk. Thanks for finding the time to be with our students."

As we walked toward the auditorium, I asked Beth about mental health issues on campus. "We have a number of students here who are having a hard time," she said. "Our counseling office is pretty busy."

I was curious. "What do you see most often?" I asked.

"A lot of kids come to see us about their anxiety and depression," she replied. "Sometimes they are in bad shape. But there are other issues, too. There is a lot of pressure on kids these days," she told me, "and some kids have a harder time dealing with it."

This school had several hundred students but was one-sixth the size of my hometown high school where we had just one guidance counselor: Mr. Dwyer. Always distinguished in his suit and tie, Mr. Dwyer was a wonderful man if you could gather the courage to talk with him, but he was not exactly approachable. He did his best to get you into a college just a notch higher than you were thinking of or, in some cases, a notch lower if your expectations didn't match your transcript, but he was supportive in every way he knew how. But I am sure he had no training in mental health counseling and nobody would ever have suggested that he should. In my high school, mental health issues didn't exist whether they existed or not. And the unwritten code of silence was honored by everyone. Kids might act out or talk back to a teacher or be truant or bully weaker kids, but they were called out for their behavior and branded with it. No one went deeper than what we could see.

As Beth and I pulled open the front doors to the new two-story white clapboard building housing the auditorium, students were streaming past us. I learned that attendance at my talk was mandatory. That builds an audience for sure, but when choice is gone, more is expected. As we were walking down a side corridor to get to the well of the auditorium, she said casually, "I can't recall if I told you when we initially spoke about getting you here, but this day is part of parents' weekend. Most parents will arrive later today," she told me, "but several are already here so don't be surprised if you see adults in the audience." I had spoken to parents and I had spoken to students but never at the same time and never at a private school. Maybe these parents would wonder why I was speaking here at all because acceptance at a school like this was a ticket to success. Maybe the students would be reluctant to open up to me or to come forward to talk if parents, maybe even their own parents, were in the audience.

Beth took me to a front-row seat while she attended to last-minute details allowing me to gather my thoughts as the auditorium began to fill up. The headmaster had made it as promised and sat just a few rows away. I respected that he came not yet knowing my message. When Beth introduced me, I stood to polite applause and then turned to speak. She had been right about the parents. There were numerous couples spread throughout the semi-circular auditorium. But it was largely students.

My talk went well and the parents seemed to be paying close attention. None looked irritated or upset by my remarks. I had made a point to watch them as unobtrusively as I could while I spoke. I had watched juries for years during closing arguments so I was pretty adept at reading faces and body language. Several parents stood with the kids to applaud when I finished. Now, I thought, would come the acid test for the students. I believed that few, if any, would dare approach me—not here and not now, especially with parents in the auditorium. Besides, I believed these kids must be pretty resilient and steadfastly secure. They were, after all, more mature than I would have been at their age heading off to a high school states or even a coast away where they would know no one upon arrival. I didn't think I could have done that in the ninth grade but all of these kids had. I admired that. I said my goodbyes to Beth and to the headmaster who came forward to thank me. When I turned to head out the side exit by the stage, I was struck by the number of students queuing up. I stayed for an additional 50 minutes. I hugged most of the two dozen students who wanted to talk. Some were in tough straights and a few almost couldn't talk. The first young girl in line was a sophomore who told me her name was Stephanie. She was with her roommate, Anne. "We roomed together as freshmen,"

Anne said softly. They had met on campus and came from different states. Home for both was a good distance away. They both looked so young and so distressed. It was early afternoon on an otherwise beautiful spring day. But not for them it wasn't. As Stephanie began to speak, the tears that I noticed building in her eyes were now streaming down her face. It was alarming to see how upset she was. "Thanks for being here today," Stephanie said, now sobbing. She then stopped. It was as if she couldn't remember what she wanted to say.

"Why are you so upset?" I asked gently trying to give her time to compose herself. Silence and tears followed.

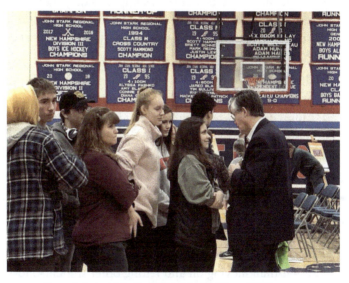

Eager students at John Stark High School in Weare, NH, line up to speak with John after his talk. (Photo credit: Margaret Haskett)

After a few painful seconds passed, she spoke like she was almost out of breath. "I have so many expectations on my back," she forced out between sobs. "I can't deal with all of it." I had never met Stephanie before this moment, but suddenly I felt committed to her well-being.

"You look like you could use a hug. Would you like one?" I asked to both distract her and let her know that I understood her pain. Rather than answer, Stephanie moved a half step closer and began hugging me. I rubbed her back for a few seconds until she gently pushed back to talk. But she couldn't get the words out.

"Stephanie," I said to her while holding both her elbows, "you wouldn't be at a school like this if you weren't pretty smart. You're going to do just fine in life. The fact you were admitted here is impressive. I don't think at your age I could have made the cut. To be honest, I stopped taking math after my sophomore year because I was so bad at it. But I've still done OK, and I know you are smarter than I was." That drew a grudging smile from her blotchy face. "Have you talked to a counselor here?"

"No," she said sadly.

"I think it would be a really good idea to do that," I told her. "I am sure they can help you. I met the head counselor today and she seemed like she really cared about all the students here. I know she can help you. Will you do that for me and reach out to her today?" I asked.

She hesitated. "I will," she told me. "I will." I hugged her.

"You're as smart as I thought you were," I told her. "Thanks for being so honest with me."

Rather than moving on and letting other students move up in the makeshift line, Stephanie and Anne were motionless. I heard Anne faintly crying. She had been a silent sentry for her friend Stephanie but it was clear she wanted to talk, too. But she couldn't speak. Literally. Anne was trying to form words as her roommate rubbed her back but she wasn't able to. Tears were pouring down her face. I asked Anne a few questions, hoping I could get her focus but to no avail. She was just distraught so I hugged her. I told Anne that she and Stephanie should see the counselor together before they left the auditorium so they could arrange a visit. Anne nodded in agreement but said nothing. She hugged me briefly and then they moved on—at least now, I hoped, with a purpose.

I learned later from Beth that Anne and Stephanie had come to see her after my visit. She confided that my talk had given Anne the courage to call her parents to let them know she needed a break from school. Apparently, the parents were going to intervene on her behalf but now didn't need to. As young as she was, Anne had taken ownership. I was so proud of her and relieved for her parents.

Several other students I spoke to that afternoon were not the usual suspects either. Three of the young men who waited to talk with me were apparently star athletes at the school. Two of them had wet eyes while we spoke, our heads but a foot apart and our eyes locked, and all three hugged me when our impromptu discussions ended. Depression, anxiety, pressure to do or be more than they thought they could and uncertainty plagued these kids. When I got to my car that afternoon to head home, I read an email from Beth, sent just a few minutes earlier. She informed me that in the hour that passed since I finished my talk, she had received 10 requests from students to come to see her. She was very appreciative. Her note said that she had never seen male students hug anyone like they were hugging me, especially varsity male athletes. I responded to her wonderful message, "When those boys were hugging me, they weren't athletes. They were just hurting."

I sat in my car for several minutes digesting my two

hours on campus. My mission seemed even more urgent than when I arrived.

I BEGAN my day pretty early the next morning. After tossing my hastily repacked bag in my Jeep and scraping a thin coating of ice from my windshield, I headed north for 90 minutes. Siri, who was indispensable to my work, was my only companion. A half-hour into the drive, there were almost no cars ahead of me on the winding interstate and just an occasional few behind. Vermont on a weekday in early April, I thought. I almost had the road to myself. The landscape I passed that frigid morning was dotted with large white farmhouses and weathered barns nestled on the brown, still frozen hillsides. Green wouldn't make its return for many more weeks; when it did, it would kick-start spring rhythms on these farms. The panoramic view from my windshield was a match for any Currier and Ives print. It was clear to me why Vermonters loved it here and why the tourists came, but I was sure the economics were difficult this far north. The rigor, sacrifices and loneliness this life demanded no doubt made it hard to get the next generation to stay. But it was sure serene and enticing on this cold spring morning.

The rural high school I pulled into that day was my furthermost stop in northern Vermont. This outpost region even had a special name: the Northeast Kingdom. It sounded very freeing to me. It seemed a really long trip for a 40-minute talk, but I was happy to be there because attending a high school just 60 miles south of Montreal likely meant these kids didn't hear from many people they didn't already know or know about. It also seemed a great opportunity to test the reception these kids might give me. Maybe, I thought, in a bucolic setting like this, the kids faced fewer challenges and would be less likely to suffer the near-epidemic anxiety and depression I found in larger, more populated school districts. Maybe the kids would sit silently when my talk ended not quite certain why I was bothering them. That would be awkward but I would soon enough find out.

When I buzzed into the school a few minutes before 9:00 a.m., the principal was happy to see me. "I thought you might not find us," he said with a smile of relief.

"I probably wouldn't have, but Siri is never wrong. Thank God for satellites," I replied. "I'm relieved to be on time. It's just starting to spit snow." Pressed for time, the principal and I walked briskly to the auditorium. During our short walk, he briefed me on the students and the towns they served.

On this day, the former Attorney General of Vermont, TJ Donovan, was joining me and would speak as he had done a half dozen other times on my visits to high schools throughout his state. He had arrived before me this morning. TJ was in his mid-40s, had been a county prosecutor and a few years earlier had been elected as Vermont's Attorney General. He spoke with a kind voice, in a gentle and thoughtful manner and with an open heart. He was totally transparent, and the students always sensed that. They knew he was here for them. I had been impressed with TJ from the first moment I met him months earlier in a high school gym in Hanover, New Hampshire, where I was scheduled to speak. He had asked to say a few words when I finished. He would speak today about someone he knew years earlier who suffered from mental health and substance misuse challenges that had really impacted his life. His remarks were always a highlight for me, and the students always listened intensely when he spoke. He would acknowledge that when he was growing up, almost no one spoke about mental illness because it was seen as a shameful weakness. I was older than TJ but I had grown up in the same culture. He would tell the students that he had been ashamed of his friend growing up, but that he was now ashamed of himself for ever feeling that way. He talked openly about the pain he had experienced watching someone he cared about suffer. It was obvious to everyone in the room that his friend's journey had touched TJ profoundly. His remarks about wiping away the shame and stigma surrounding mental illness were acutely personal and deeply felt.

You could have heard a pin drop when he spoke. No one ever expected an attorney general to come to their high school and share personal painful memories to benefit them. But TJ did it with genuine humility and grace. His remarks always paved the way for my message about starting a new conversation about mental illness without shame, blame or stigma.

The students were in their seats and waiting when the principal and I walked down one of the carpeted aisles to the front of the room. The well-appointed amphitheater auditorium was surprisingly modern with well-spaced seats in generous elevated rows. The seats were filled, and numerous students and teachers stood looking down at us from open corridors along both sides of the amphitheater. It was a full house of perfect strangers like so many I had stood before in countless other schools during the previous two years. But if things went as I hoped, the barriers between us would drop by the time I finished speaking, and I would get to share hugs and stories with kids I didn't know and would never likely see again. That's why I had come. That's what sustained me on long days. But this far north, in surroundings as bucolic and tranquil as these, I wasn't sure that would be the case.

After the students quieted down, the principal took the mic from its stand. "It is an honor to have Chief Justice Broderick here today to talk with all of us about mental health," he said. "I expect you will give him your full attention. Please give him a warm Vermont welcome." The kids were still applauding as he walked over to pass me the mic.

Mic in hand, I walked to the well of the auditorium. I was just a few feet from the students in the front row. The room fell quiet. I never stood on a stage in rooms like this because I wanted to be on the same level as the kids. I wasn't there to give them a lecture. I just wanted to talk with them about my family's journey with mental illness, my ignorance and the mistakes I made. Standing close to them made that easier and more personal. I wanted to shrink the room. I was there to share what I had learned and seen these last few years from students, teachers and counselors in rooms like this. But mostly, above all, I wanted to give them hope. I wanted them to know that if they or someone they loved had a mental health problem, they were not alone and that treatment was possible.

I began my talk that morning as I always did. "I came here this morning because I need your help. That's why I'm at your high school today," I told them. That got their attention. "I'm a baby boomer," I confessed, "not that you could have ever guessed that." Students almost always smiled when I said that. I'm sure I looked like a grandfather they had never met. "When I was your age and for much of my adult life," I continued, "people never talked about mental illness. It just wasn't a conversation people were willing to have. Mental illness was always viewed as a weakness, a character flaw or a failing of some sort, so no one mentioned it. No one. I was so ignorant about it that I didn't even see it for what it was when it took up residence in my 13-year-old son. Ignorance helps no one," I told them, "and it almost destroyed my family." They were all listening now. No telltale light from iPhone screens was visible anywhere. The students were listening.

"We need to change the conversation around mental illness and learn what it is and what it isn't," I said. "It's a health issue and not a weakness. We need to normalize it, demythologize it, remove it from the shadows where it has been hiding for generations and finally get people the help they deserve."

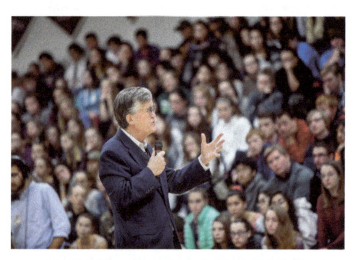

John delivers his message to a rapt crowd at Lebanon High School in New Hampshire's Upper Valley. (Photo credit: Mark Washburn)

I briefly paused but then continued. "For real change to happen, I will need your generation to help. You are the least judgmental generation in the history of the United

States. So, if change is going to happen, you need to lead it. I need your voices." With my voice rising with emotion I said, "If I could change it by myself I would, but I can't. But we could change it if you want. I have confidence that I will have your help because your generation is smarter than I was. I know your generation wants this conversation to happen. I do, too."

I spoke for almost 40 minutes, and the students barely moved. It wasn't about me, I knew that. It was about what I was saying. They weren't used to someone my age talking so openly about emotional suffering and they could relate to it. I was sure of that. One in five adolescents has a mental health challenge and they all likely had friends, neighbors or family members who were suffering, too. They got it. I recounted my family's painful story and assured them that we had come through the fire. I shared anecdotes that kids their age had shared with me in the impersonal surroundings of gyms and auditoriums scattered across northern New England just to let them know they were not alone.

As I concluded, I again appealed to them. "If you won't help me change the culture around mental health for yourself or a classmate or a family member, please help me for your own children. Most of you here will be parents one day. Some of your kids will have mental health challenges just like my own son. I know that statistically. We don't want another generation in the shadows ashamed and afraid. There is nothing to fear and there is zero shame. Treatment is possible. Silence changes nothing. I need your voices and I am confident I will have them." With that, I ended and slowly walked over to put the mic back in the stand. After a moment of dead silence, kids began to applaud and stand in small groups until the entire auditorium was standing and clapping. It was their way of affirming the message, of embracing the challenge they knew we all had to meet.

After the Attorney General spoke, students started coming forward to talk; some in groups of two or three and some alone. Most wanted to thank me for "talking about it" and others wanted to hug me and share their stories. Sometimes when they seemed upset, I would ask them if they needed a hug. No one said no. Some kids had tears in their eyes. Knowing I had a two-hour drive south for another talk at another high school that afternoon, I tried to watch the clock, but I never rushed anyone who wanted to confide; some had tough homes and tough circumstances. Many were getting help with their emotional problems but many weren't. I often suggested they talk to a counselor at their school if they were going it alone. Even when I reached the corridor adjacent to the auditorium on my way to the front entrance, kids were still stopping me to talk. I listened.

I remember one young student that day as I was inching ever closer to the exit who opened up about her anxiety and began crying. I just hugged her and encouraged her to get help. When I mentioned to her that she was not alone and that a lot of her classmates were facing similar challenges, she looked up through her wet eyes and said, "Almost everyone in this school has issues." It always amazed me how open kids were with a perfect stranger like me. But over time I began to realize they just needed to talk with someone who listened and understood. They knew I wouldn't blame them or shame them for their suffering. That's all it took. It was almost noon by the time I said goodbye to the principal. "In this storm," he said, "you'll be lucky to arrive on time for your next talk." I left in a hurry and walked as fast as I could to my car that was now coated with snow.

When I finally arrived just before 2:00 p.m. at my final stop, a small high school in yet another picturesque Vermont farming community of rolling hills and fenced pastures, I had no time on the clock. I had to park and be in the auditorium in three minutes. But I was grateful to have made it in two hours, given the country roads I was traveling were slowed tremendously by an unexpected spring snowstorm. My black Jeep was streaked with frozen slush and road salt by the time I pulled into the parking lot, but I had made it.

The drive south had been a white-knuckle experience to be sure, but northern New England in early spring often made road trips dicey. Today was just a reminder. Despite the pressure and stress of my trip south that afternoon with one eye on the clock and the other on snowy roads, I couldn't stop replaying the images and stories of the kids I had hugged and encouraged just a few hours earlier. They came with me. They always came with me.

Somehow, I managed to begin my second talk of the day just a few minutes after 2:00 p.m. It was another full auditorium of students, only now their day would be over as soon as my talk ended. I wondered whether anyone would pay attention now because this likely seemed like a throw-away period before they boarded the buses. But again, they listened. They were silent and focused. Nobody was fooling around in that cavernous room with the 30-foot ceiling; no teachers were rustling to caution students about their behavior. I spoke to them as I had spoken more than 200 times before on days that now seemed to blur together. But I drew energy from the kids each time I spoke. We connected; their attention let me know they recognized my effort. After almost 45 minutes, I concluded my talk. It came none too soon as my voice was beginning to sound a bit hoarse. The kids stood and warmly applauded. I was exhausted and looking forward to getting to my car and heading home. I had a long drive ahead of me in the snow. And then the students started lining up to talk. It surprised me how many kids waited—they weren't missing classes so there was no incentive to stay behind.

After 75 minutes of very personal conversations with hurting kids, I noticed there was one student left. He was sitting in the front row of the now dimly lit auditorium. It was almost 4:00 p.m. "Did you want to see me?" I asked. Quite honestly, I was drained after my long day of driving and speaking, and I was hoping he had just been waiting for a friend.

"If I can," he said passively. He had waited patiently for a long time. I walked a few paces toward him and he stood. We were alone except for a school counselor sitting in the last row of the auditorium. But she couldn't hear us. He was heavyset and fairly tall. He told me his first name. "What year are you in?" I asked.

"I'm a junior," he replied softly. He looked sad to me like someone who felt forgotten.

"How are you doing?" I asked him. He then began to open up to me. I heard about his family and the dysfunction he lived in every day. I heard how he had few friends. His eyes began to tear up. "Are you seeing anyone about all you're dealing with?" I asked him. "What's going on in your life would be hard for anyone to sort through." I couldn't ask him to talk with his parents since by his account they were at the root of his unhappiness.

"No," he said forlornly. Then silence ensued.

"Maybe you should talk to one of the counselors here at school. They could help you," I suggested. He was looking right at me but I could tell he hadn't heard me. He was now crying, his face only inches from mine. I put my hand firmly on his shoulder.

"Can I tell you something?" he asked with some urgency.

"Sure, what?" I replied.

"I'm thinking of killing myself, and I even know where I'm going to do it and how." Tears were rolling down his cheeks. I gently grabbed his elbows.

"No, we're not doing that," I heard myself say. "That's not who YOU are. That's what's bothering who you are. That's your depression, and we can deal with that. You seem like such a great guy. I feel so badly about all you are dealing with. None of that is your fault. I hope you know that. It would be hard for anyone. I want you to see the counselor before I leave. She's in the back of the auditorium. Will you promise me you will do that?"

"I will," he whispered.

"Is that a commitment? I couldn't tell."

"Yes," he said more affirmatively, "I promise." He then hugged me like someone he knew but hadn't seen for years.

"I'm proud of you," I told him. "Thanks so much for waiting all the time you did to talk with me." I walked him up the aisle to the counselor. "This young man is having a real hard time. Not his fault. He promised me he would tell you what we shared." He smiled at me. "I promise," he said.

By the time I got to my car, I was drained and emotionally spent. I was happy that I had not ducked out of that last meeting with that young man, claiming that I had a long trip ahead of me. I was thankful I had been at his school on this day and that he was brave enough to trust me. As I headed south at the end of another long day, I knew I could not have had a more important conversation with anyone on earth that afternoon. I knew my mission mattered. I hoped that young man got the help he deserved.

I HAD SPOKEN at the high school in this New Hampshire town months earlier. It had gone well. The principal there stood out. He seemed way ahead of the curve on mental health. The students had really responded to my message that winter morning that I spoke, and I hugged and talked with several kids when my remarks were over.

The high school was state-of-the-art and surrounded by acres of lush playing fields and expansive parking. It was home to more than 700 kids. You could almost feel the expectations those kids brought with them every morning in their backpacks and athletic bags. Many came from the newly wealthy families who had been moving into town over the last 10 years. Everyone had plans for these kids. Many kids embraced those ambitions and were competing to achieve all they could, but some of the kids I spoke with were feeling crushed under the weight of plans that were largely the dreams of others. Those kids had shared their anxieties with me. I remembered their faces.

But this day, I would not be returning to the high school but would be speaking at the middle school of 300 kids in grades six through eight. I was feeling more comfortable giving my talk to middle schoolers by this point, although I was always surprised and humbled by the attention they paid. "If I were here to talk to kids about the courts and government, many of their eyes would glaze over," I had told many middle school principals these last several months. But talking about mental health almost always got the kids' full focus. This March morning the principal had assembled all the kids in the gym for my 8:30 a.m. talk.

When the principal and I entered the gym, I noticed that the sixth- and seventh-graders sat on the gym floor while the more privileged eighth-graders got the bleachers. I pointed that out to the younger kids on the floor. "Just another reminder that life is not fair," I said. Many of the kids smiled. I had broken the ice. Even though they had to be uncomfortable sitting cross-legged on the shiny gym floor, once I began my talk they were intently listening to my story. I quickly forgot their ages. They understood and oddly I understood them. Although I knew that for them, growing up in a post-9/11 world was much harder than what I experienced in the comparatively slower-paced world of the late 1950s, I always sensed they were stronger and smarter than I had been. So, despite the mounting challenges of their childhood beyond the walls of their school, I hoped they would persevere and change what needed changing. They had experienced way more of the real world than I had at their age. When I finished, the kids, without prompting, began to applaud. A few gave me wide smiles, and a few had wet eyes. We had connected across the decades that divided us.

As the kids were leaving the gym to begin their regular school routines, I stood by the exit with their principal watching them parade past. Some spoke in quick bursts ("loved your story," "great talk") as they passed in swarms and some offered clipped "thank yous." But near the end of the exodus was a young boy with an outstretched right hand. I shook it reflexively. I was thinking as I felt his soft hand in mine that I would never have had his courage and poise when I was his young age. He promptly told me that he was 13 and in the eighth grade. "Thanks for coming to my school this morning and talking about this," he said.

"Oh, I was more than happy to come," I replied. "All of you seemed to be listening. I really appreciated that." He remained just a foot away from me with his small hand still firmly in mine.

"I want to tell you why I'm thanking you," he said with more than a bit of emotion in his voice.

"Sure," I replied, "why?"

"They tell me at school that I'm on the spectrum," he said, referring to autism spectrum disorder. He paused slightly and took a breath. His eyes were moist. "Your talk here this morning has changed my whole life," he said. "Can I hug you?" He quickly ended our handshake to put both of his thin arms around my waist and began to cry. "Thanks for being here," he said. My eyes began to water, too. After a quick final tight squeeze, he let go suddenly and was swept away into the final flow of students leaving the gym.

As I was driving away from the school that morning, I knew I hadn't changed that boy's life, but I thought that maybe for the first time in his young life, he found the courage to share his challenges with a perfect stranger who he knew would not judge him or blame him for his difficulties. My visit had mattered to him. That much was certain. That was reward enough.

I WAS LOOKING FORWARD to speaking to the school kids in the working-class, no-pretense New Hampshire town where my youngest son lived and worked for a couple of years after he graduated from college. He had loved the place and its people. Everybody seemed to know everybody else. The town was mostly hard-working blue collar, although there was a small but growing number of professionals moving in. Increasingly, more residents drove south to Massachusetts to work every morning, although there was still a well-worn path north to Concord and Manchester. Its downtown was home to small shops, restaurants, convenience marts, a few chain drugstores and the ever-present gas stations.

But the town had no public high school of its own. It sent its ninth-graders to the high school in the larger, more prosperous neighboring town or sometimes to the campus-like semi-private high school at the edge of town. But every kid passed through the middle schools in town. In fact, the town had two—one a bit newer and a bit more upscale than the other—but both a source of pride for the townspeople. Between them, their enrollment exceeded 1,000 kids in grades six through eight. I had spoken in town more than a year earlier at the invitation of the school superintendent, but it was an evening event focused on talking to parents about mental health awareness. About 300 people came out that night, and there was a nice story in the local paper. But today's visit would be different. I would be talking to almost 600 middle school kids.

As I turned into the school parking lot, I noticed a small group of uniformed police officers striding toward the school's front entrance. My first reaction was that something dreadful must have happened, but when I saw kids being dropped off and rushing past the officers into the building, I thought maybe the officers were coming to hear my talk. I knew of their chief and his interest in mental health. Maybe he had "ordered" them to come. Whatever the reason, I was grateful they were there. I had learned in my work that more police and first responders died by suicide each year than died from all other causes in the line of duty combined. Nobody ever talked about that nasty little secret, but the police were beginning to soften to the discussion. All of us needed to. Their presence in the gym when the kids began assembling for my talk would not go unnoticed. I needed allies in the awareness campaign, and local police in small-town New Hampshire were well-liked, well-known and admired. They could be invaluable. Today was a great opportunity to see if I could secure their support.

Things got underway on time. The kids streamed into the gym by class. The sixth- and seventh-graders took the folding metal chairs laid out across the floor, and the eighth-graders got the bleachers. There were a number of teachers and a few members of the school board in the audience. Even the police chief was there. The principal introduced me, and when I stood to take the mic, the background hum from the students stopped. The huge room fell quiet.

The kids listened—really listened for 40 minutes. I always regretted that parents weren't there to see the attention kids paid to a topic that still made most adults uncomfortable. I wasn't sure how this young crowd, a third of whom were 10 or 11 years old, would react when my talk ended. I closed as I always did by asking for their help to start a new conversation around mental illness. I asked them to join me to eliminate the shame and stigma that had hurt too many people for way too long. The silence was soon broken as the kids began to applaud and stand, led by the sixth-graders in the front of the room. When I was in the sixth grade, I knew I wouldn't have stood. I likely would have been bored. I wouldn't have related to what I was telling them. Not these kids. Their enthusiastic response told me they understood.

After the principal dismissed them, a young girl, a sixth-grader, moved forward toward me as her classmates were leaving. She was blonde, slight and wearing a very sad face. "Thank you for speaking here today," she said so softly that I strained to hear her. She looked like she wanted to say more but seemed overwhelmed.

"How are you doing?" I asked just to keep the conversation alive.

"Not that well," she replied. "I feel very sad and depressed. I'm thinking of killing myself." It was stunning to hear that cry for help from her angelic face. I instinctively hugged her and she squeezed me back.

"Oh, my goodness," I heard myself say, "that can't be the answer. Nothing can be that bad. I'm sure you feel terrible about something or maybe a lot of things, but people can help you with all of that. You can never give up on yourself," I said trying to convince her. She told me her name was Morgan. We talked for a few minutes in the now empty gym: two strangers of greatly different ages that fate had brought together in a very unlikely place. Things were not great at home for her and school had become stressful, too. I asked her if she was talking to a teacher or counselor at school about how she was feeling.

"I'm not," Morgan said.

"Well, I want you to," I quickly replied. "You seem like a very special girl and I don't want you to be this unhappy." She looked up at me with sad eyes. She said nothing. "Do you know what a pinkie promise is?" I asked her.

"Yes, I do."

"Those are the ones you can't break, right?" I asked her.

"I never break those promises," she declared.

"Good," I said with a smile, "how about making a pinkie promise with me?"

She nodded her head to agree. I hooked my right little finger and extended it toward her. I was now bending down. She seemed so small. She extended her fragile pinkie to meet mine. Her hand was dwarfed by mine. We hooked fingers. "Here's the promise I want you to make," I told her. She was looking into my eyes. "I want you to see a counselor or teacher today before school is over and tell them exactly what you told me. Will you pinkie promise you will do that today?" I asked her. She didn't hesitate.

"I will," she said. "I promise."

"Thank you," I told her as she ran to catch up to her classmates. "I'm counting on you." Then she was gone.

As I stood reflecting on what had just happened, I heard the principal's voice. "Judge Broderick, can you stay for lunch?" She asked as she walked toward me across the gym. "I think the kids would really enjoy that if you have time."

"Happy to," I said, although I felt spent. The previous day had been a long one with a lot of time on the road between talks, but it was not the type of invitation I could really decline. She explained that they had six 22-minute lunch shifts with 100 kids per shift. "They begin eating lunch at 10:30?" I asked, thinking I clearly must have misunderstood her.

"Pretty close," she replied. "Our cafeteria space is somewhat limited but the kids have adapted to it. You might be able to sit down for a few minutes," she said. "Maybe a few students will want to talk with you."

"Sure, I can do that," I responded. "Sitting down is pretty appealing right now, and a cold drink sounds great."

As we entered the cafeteria, the first lunch shift was just arriving. Kids were scurrying everywhere trying to find seats with friends and some were trading treats in their lunch bags. Their many voices created a din. I felt very old and awkwardly out of place in their world of familiarity. Everyone knew everyone in this room. They had been friends and classmates through grade school with many of the same memories of classrooms, teachers, field trips and countless other things that shaped their young lives. Whatever they had done, they had essentially done it together.

They were the world for each other. And the teachers monitoring the cafeteria were larger than life to these kids, too. I was sure of that. I remembered that much from my middle school days. But I was the only true stranger in the room. I was the only one who seemed out of place. The kids had heard me speak and had been surprisingly gracious, but this place and these 22 minutes were theirs. I doubted they would share it. I expected it might be a lonely shift before I could quietly exit.

As I looked for a place to sit, I felt a tap on my back. I turned to find a girl with brown shoulder-length hair looking up at me. "Thanks for your story," she said. "I have a story, too." Her brown eyes looked bottomless.

"What's your story?" I inquired.

"I'm new to this school and I don't have many friends," she said in a clipped manner as if to preface what she really wanted to tell me.

"That's hard, isn't it?" I replied. "When I was in the fourth grade, my family moved and I had to go to a new school where I didn't know anybody. But I made friends there and you will, too. Just be patient with yourself."

"Can I tell you something else?" she asked.

"Of course," I replied.

She was now looking down. "I was molested by my stepfather, and I am feeling really depressed and anxious."

Stunned and unprepared for this revelation, I immediately hugged her. She squeezed me back. "That's not your fault. You know that, right?" I asked her.

"Yes," she said softly. Worried that law enforcement had not been involved, I asked if the assault had been reported to the police. It had, she assured me. He had been arrested. But reported or not, she was suffering its devastating impact. She was in middle school.

"Are you talking with a counselor about how you are feeling?" I asked. I couldn't begin to imagine how she was dealing with everything. I had heard several sexual assault appeals as a judge but I had never hugged a victim. She was just a kid. I was angry for her.

"I had a counselor in my other school and I just got a new one here," she said.

"That's exactly what you should be doing," I told her. "You should be proud of how brave you are." I so wanted to give her her childhood back but another hug and heartfelt encouragement were all I could offer. I just hoped she could get the help she needed to begin to sort it out but feared it would likely steal her adolescence and more. I felt so helpless. Then she disappeared into the jumble of the lunchroom. I remember her still.

I talked with so many middle school students that day in the cafeteria that I never got a chance to even sit down until the fifth lunch period. The students queued up single file or with a friend just to talk and share. Some gave me art they had drawn to thank me for coming and many gave me hugs. I gladly returned them. I heard about anxiety, depression, bipolar disorder, problems at home, divorces gone terribly wrong, drugs and alcoholism. The kids shared so openly. They were so courageous and trusting. I had never been a part of their lives until that morning but they welcomed me in. Most often the stories I heard were about their own suffering, but sometimes it was about the witnessed suffering of others they loved or knew and wanted so desperately to help. I even hugged a few kids that day who had tried to kill themselves. One eighth-grade boy shared in hushed tones that he had twice tried to end his own life. The school knew his story, he told me, and he was getting help from a counselor.

After more than an hour and a half of standing on a hard cafeteria floor and engaging dozens and dozens of kids, I felt that I needed a break. I needed time away from the suffering just to process all I had heard. Half the students who confided in me were not getting any help or at least not enough. Some told me they were ashamed. So, when a lull came between shifts, I took it. I invited myself to sit at a nearby table of eighth-grade girls who had just arrived for their 22-minute lunch. They were busy unwrapping, unpacking and talking with each other when I interrupted their bubble of privacy.

"Do you guys mind if I join you?" I asked. I was uncertain how they might react and I was sure I would not have been their table's first choice. But with no time to confer, they were at a distinct disadvantage.

"Sure, have a seat," one of the girls said with a bit of uncertainty in her voice. Because the die had been cast, the others followed suit and welcomed me to their table.

After a few awkward moments, I was able to get them talking. After getting a handle on who they were and what their interests were, I asked, "Do you guys have iPhones?"

"Of course," was their refrain colored with a tinge of disbelief that I would think for a second that they were not tech-savvy. They all had them. I was curious how much time they spent on them every day, although I didn't think they would give me the real number. But I asked anyway. Several girls said, "four or five hours." When I asked how much of that related to schoolwork, the estimates were all south of 40 minutes. One girl seemed reticent to say anything. "How about you?" I asked her. "How much time do you spend on your phone?"

"I only use mine for maybe an hour or two a day," she said apologetically.

"That's very good," I told her. "How come you're on your phone much less than everyone else is?"

She hesitated for a moment, "To be honest," she replied, "if I use it more than an hour or two a day, I get depressed." I was sure that was a painful confession. I admired her honesty. But she was by no means alone. Social media has contributed to a real spike in teenage depression and anxiety in America. The virtual world, as essential as it is, can be a difficult space to navigate alone for impressionable kids who are often made to feel different, shortchanged, left out or undervalued on its screens. Snapchat, Instagram and TikTok are a world unto themselves—a world where kids can get lost, confused and misled. I wasn't sorry I grew up without them.

As my time at the table was coming to a close, I asked my lunchmates if it was true that their generation felt really stressed. Almost immediately the girl to my right exclaimed, "We are!" Everyone at the table was nodding along in agreement. Some were smiling as if I had finally asked them the right question.

"Why is that?" I asked.

"We are always trying to accomplish the next thing so we can be eligible for the thing after that. That causes real stress," she said with authority, "real stress."

Another chimed in, "I freak out if I don't get a 100 on every paper." After 15 minutes of surprisingly open conversation, the kids at my table got ready to head out to their next class. A few pulled books from their knapsacks while others scanned their phones as if looking for urgent messages. I was sorry my time with them was ending. Despite my initial reservations, I had really enjoyed them. They made me feel included and rewarded me with their simple honesty. Age and awkwardness had melted away.

This generation of kids was different for sure. They were more open and informed than I had been in middle school, but they were also more stressed and anxious, living in a more demanding, competitive and anonymous world than I ever experienced. "Thanks for coming today," several of the girls said as they rose to be on their way.

As I was thanking them for letting me crash their lunch, I noticed the girl I had hugged just two hours earlier in the gym striding purposely toward me with a tall, fair-skinned, middle-aged woman at her side. I stood to greet them.

"Good to see you again," I said to Morgan.

The woman put her hand lightly on Morgan's shoulders as if to give her a cue. "Morgan has something she wants to tell you," the woman informed me.

"Remember I made a pinkie promise to you in the gym," she said triumphantly.

"I do remember," I replied smiling.

"Well, I kept it. She's the counselor," Morgan said proudly, looking up at her companion. She had wasted no time completing her mission. It was like a hunting dog that had retrieved the downed bird.

"I'm really proud of you," I said. "You're just as smart and strong as I thought you were." Morgan hugged me quickly and then ran back to join her table. I introduced myself to the counselor and we began chatting.

As we were shaking hands she confided, "We usually know who the kids are that are struggling but we didn't know about Morgan." She paused. "But we know now." Morgan had apparently stopped her in the stairwell on her way to lunch just a few minutes earlier. "She asked if she could come to see me," the counselor said. "She told me that she promised you she would see someone today. She wanted you to know that she kept her promise."

As I was leaving the cafeteria a few minutes later, I was still talking to the kids who approached me. They were still sharing and confiding. I had never experienced anything like it. Days like these were challenging me and making me even more impatient to rally the larger community to listen, to learn and to act. I felt a kinship with these kids who entrusted me with their stories and their fears. I was wishing I could return the next day to continue learning from them. There seemed so much more to do.

ONE SPRING MORNING with temperatures still fluttering in the low 40s, I pulled into the parking lot at a middle school a few miles inland on the Maine coast. The school was an older two-story red brick building with a mismatched addition located a stone's throw from neighborhoods of modest clapboard houses. Its setting reminded me of the grade school I had attended as a child.

Although I had visited several middle schools by then, I was still a bit anxious about the reaction of sixth-, seventh- and eighth-graders to my talk. I couldn't shake the uneasiness. I was, after all, more than five decades older than my audience that morning and had been shaped, comforted, enriched and sometimes challenged by a world they would never experience. But that same world that nurtured me had kept mental health awareness off my radar and everyone's radar as best I could remember. The world I came from had been bold enough to talk about civil rights, religious bigotry and sexual freedom, but had steered clear of mental health. I understood now that the bubble of silence I grew up in had left me shortchanged and unprepared to spot mental illness when it entered my own home and took up residence in my own son. He was about the age of these kids when it entered his life. I knew statistically that some of the kids I would be speaking to that morning were silently suffering as my son had while thinking their discomfort was "just them." Maybe they were too afraid or self-conscious to reach out or speak up. Maybe there was no language for their feelings. Maybe their parents were as clueless as we had been.

The kids were walking and running past me, talking and laughing on their way to the gym when I walked through the front door. The principal was there to welcome me as she had promised. After hanging up my coat in the office and greeting the few staff, I followed the principal down the main corridor bedecked with student art. The echoes and murmurs of young voices coming toward us from the gym were unexpectedly soothing. The principal was surprisingly candid about the mental health challenges some of the kids were facing. But there was no time for me to probe further and ask questions.

The gym was timeless. The polished bleachers standing tall against opposite walls had not been opened. The wooden floor was glistening, and two basketball nets with glass backboards hung awkwardly at odd angles above the floor. There were even a few championship banners hanging from the beige 30-foot walls. The kids were seated in metal folding chairs laid out in precise rows on black runners. Their young faces were not confidence builders. I was, after all, a perfect stranger to them and much older than their parents. They were all perfect strangers to me, too.

A few teachers walked over to thank me for coming as I stood just inside the doorway waiting for the principal to introduce me. This was always the moment when self-doubt crept in. No matter how many times I had given my talk, I couldn't shake the disquieting feeling that the kids might not listen to me for more than a few polite minutes before being distracted by friends or iPhones. That hadn't been my experience anywhere to date, but it was always a risk. It was, I suppose, the fear of revealing myself in such a personal way to strangers two generations younger who might wonder why I was bothering them. What if I was describing the unimaginable parts of our descent into despair and hopelessness and saw kids laughing or fooling around? How would I react? How would I continue my talk without feeling that I was devaluing my son's suffering or betraying his courage?

My story was intended to open minds, begin a long-delayed discussion and allow those suffering and those who loved them to experience hope. I was on a mission of change. Young people represented my only real hope to drive that change. They were much less afraid. I needed their voices and impatience, and I needed to inspire them to join me. I was not there for entertainment value or to fill a free period. Every time I spoke, I relived our nightmare and depleted myself. I just wanted it to be worth it. But when my talk and personal visits with kids were over, as tired as I felt, I had always been comforted by the stories and hugs that kids so willingly shared. Their gifts of candor and vulnerability sustained me through long days. Change always seemed more urgent to me in those incomparable moments —and more possible, too.

When the principal finished her gracious introduction, she passed the hand mic to me and joined her colleagues standing along the wall. The students quietly applauded as if uncertain as to who I was, why I was there or what I might say. They seemed so incredibly young and innocent. As I began my talk, it was hard to imagine that any of them were suffering from anxiety, depression or stress of any kind. I remembered what the principal had shared as we were walking to the gym, but I would never have believed it looking at these kids. Their faces brought me back to my own memories of what junior high felt like and of my own family and childhood during those years.

Back then, I had felt secure, loved and able to deal with whatever angst was typical for a young teenager growing up in a middle-class town. The mental illness that almost destroyed my family much later had been invisible to me at their age. Maybe, I thought, it was invisible to them, too. But the statistics belied that. As I shared my story and made my plea for them to help me change the shameful culture around mental illness, they were not disengaged but riveted. It was stunning. They understood what I never even saw in my childhood. The statistics were revealing themselves in the faces in front of me as I spoke. A few kids were emotional, and one student got up and walked from the gym. I later learned that she had a member of her own family afflicted with serious mental illness. It had been hard for her to listen.

Talking with those kids that morning and seeing them listening—really listening—gave me hope that my message would resonate beyond my visit. Maybe all they needed was a new vocabulary to speak about their emotional struggles and the long-withheld permission to describe them openly without shame or fear of being judged. Both were essential for change to happen. That much I knew.

As my talk ended, I saw a few kids wiping tears from their cheeks. They were all standing now and applauding. I felt a part of them as I made eye contact with their young faces. I felt connected to their struggles. I had been in their school less than an hour and managed to break down the generational barrier between us with my own story. I just hoped it would free them to share their stories, and if not with me, then with a parent, friend or teacher. Someone. I knew from experience that speaking your pain was essential to moving ahead. Real progress demanded awkward moments and trust. I had somehow formed a bond with those kids who I now knew were stronger, smarter and more at risk than I had been when I sat in their chairs decades earlier. I felt the relief that comes from making a real, personal connection.

As if rehearsed, the principal stepped forward to congratulate the kids on the courtesy they had shown me while encouraging them to give me one more round of applause. As the clapping subsided, she told them, "You should head now to your next scheduled period. But," she quickly added, "if you want to talk to Judge Broderick, he will be here for another 15 minutes or so." At that invitation, chairs began to move and kids began to disperse. I expected no one would likely have the time or courage to talk. Many kids moved quickly to the exit, but others began to queue up in front of me.

By the time the kids lined up, they must have numbered 25. I knew I would be there a lot longer than 15 minutes. They were all shapes and sizes and all seemed pretty sedate, no doubt thinking about what they would tell me. But they all had one thing in common: they were all 14 years old or younger. That stark reality was not lost on me. I thought of the courage it took for them to stand out like this in front of teachers and classmates and make very personal disclosures to someone they had never met. I wondered if their parents would be surprised if they knew their child was standing in this line. I was flooded with thoughts of my own son who had been their age once. He was suffering then, but had told me years later that he would never have had the courage at that age to share his inner self with anyone. He believed it was just him and that he would outgrow or outrun whatever it was that was making him feel different and be less than he wanted to be.

As I took the first child's perspiration-soaked outstretched hand, I wondered how many of these kids had opened up about their feelings and stresses to their parents or whether they would be sharing confidences with me that never found their way home. I also knew from both statistics and prior experience—some of it in my own family—that not every kid feeling uncomfortable in their own skin would feel comfortable sharing that.

As the first seventh-grade boy began to talk with me, I could barely hear him. He was speaking in a hushed tone. In his mind, I'm sure he thought he was about to share a monumental secret. I bent over to be close to his face so I could hear him. His brown eyes were wide and wet. "Thanks for coming here today," he whispered. "I have horrible anxiety. Some days it's hard for me to come to school. I feel alone and afraid a lot," he shared quietly. Fighting back tears he asked, "Can I give you a hug?"

"Sure," I said, as his small arms reached around me. "I love hugs. Are you talking with anyone about how you're feeling?" I asked him.

"Not really," he confided. "I've told my mom, but she tells me that I will get over it."

"Have you talked to a counselor at school?" I asked him. "You know whatever you're feeling is not your fault, right?" He nodded but it was clear that's not how he felt. "You're not the only student here who feels like you do," I assured him. "But the first step is to talk to someone who will understand.

That's what your school counselor is here for. Will you do that for me?" He nodded in agreement. "Maybe she can reach out to your mom. You haven't done anything wrong. You should be proud that you told me."

"I will talk to her if you really think it would help," he said sheepishly.

"I do." I was smiling at him now. "You promise me?" I asked as he began to move away and toward his next class.

"I will, I promise," he said. Then he was gone as quickly as he had appeared. I don't remember his name but I will never forget that wet hand.

For the next 25 minutes, the line of young faces with hard stories and damp eyes streamed past me. I hugged almost everyone I talked to. Most often, they hugged me first. I heard about tough times at home, pressures to achieve and difficulties just getting through the day. Anxiety and depression were far-too common afflictions. These fragile kids were so uncertain and so in need of assurance. They wanted my time and deserved my full attention. I tried to be totally present to each of them and hold eye contact when they would let me. It was always exhausting, but they made me feel so essential as they opened up to me and confided their pain.

Listening intently to their stories was hard to do without feeling overwhelmed. Every few minutes, it was a different kid reaching out, searching, asking, sharing. I always encouraged them to talk to their parents, but they were often hesitant. They had learned the shame we had taught them and they knew of the stigma. They didn't want to disappoint. When I sensed their reluctance to discuss their emotional distress at home, I tried to have them talk to a teacher or counselor in their school, someone they could trust. But some days it felt like I was doing triage with too little knowledge and too few resources. Looking into young, trusting eyes that were awaiting a silver-bullet answer was wrenching. I wanted to cure their problems but couldn't. Over time, I came to appreciate that just listening and affirming them and letting them know that they were not their illness, that they were not the only ones, provided long-overdue comfort.

After about 30 minutes, half a dozen kids remained. A few were talking to the kid in front of them, but most were silent, heads down. There were still a few teachers milling around the gym, and I wondered if I was hindering activities or interfering with classes. I felt a bit uncomfortable because of the unplanned length of my stay, but I decided to remain and talk with all the kids who had waited so patiently and so bravely to talk to a stranger.

As I was momentarily distracted, wondering what I would say if I were asked by a school official to cut short my talks with the waiting students, I heard a small, quiet voice. "Judge Broderick, thanks for coming today." When I snapped back to the present, I saw a slight, bespectacled young boy leaning slightly forward in his wheelchair just a foot away from my legs. It was jarring seeing someone his age dealing with such a profound disability. I couldn't imagine how he could accept his lot without anger or bitterness. Yet here he was with courage and poise I never had in the seventh grade. Here he was in this line, attracting more unwanted attention to himself. Junior high was hard enough with everyone trying to just fit in and not be noticed. His very presence announced his differences.

"Your talk meant a lot to me," he said as he looked up with his wide blue eyes. He reached his right hand up to shake mine, and I took it. "I have never heard an adult talk like that," he told me.

Because it seemed disrespectful to be towering over him, I kept hold of his hand and bent down on one knee so he and I could speak from the same level. His name was Ryan.

"How are you doing?" I asked him. "You were great to wait in this long line."

"I'm actually not doing too well," he said with an aching sadness in his voice.

It broke my heart that someone so young could be so sad. "What's happening that's making you feel so down?" I asked him.

"It's getting harder and harder to be in this wheelchair," he told me. "I have friends, and I used to be able to keep up with them, but they are walking too fast now. Many don't talk to me like they used to. I feel left out more and more," he confessed. His eyes narrowed in pain.

"That's hard, isn't it?" I replied. I couldn't imagine how challenging his life must be or how steep the mountain he climbed every day just getting through school. And his life would not be getting easier any time soon, I thought—likely harder. In just a few short years, his friends would be driving, dating, playing sports, going to parties, all things that would be difficult to do from a wheelchair. I feared adjusting to that loss would overwhelm him, intensifying his growing feelings of isolation. His friends would be moving in circles where it would be hard for him to follow; where his differences would be harder to accommodate. I could sense his fear of being abandoned and alone. His physical limitations were hard, but his emotional response to them was really weighing him down.

"It's making me feel sad and angry, too," he confided.

"Anyone who doesn't realize what a special person you are is not good enough to be your friend," I assured him. "You are an incredible young man," I told him trying to keep my eyes from watering. "I hope you know that." He smiled meekly. "But I think it would be good to talk to the counselor here at school and to share your feelings with her. Are you willing to do that?" I asked gently.

"Yes," he said quickly, "I will." He then leaned forward in his wheelchair and put his arms around my neck and squeezed. I rubbed his back. After a few seconds, he slid his arms down to the wheels of his chair. He was crying. My last image of him was seeing him spinning across the gym to the far exit. My junior high memories would not be his, but I had never had the courage he did, either.

Feeling emotionally spent, I stood to talk with the last student. He had waited a long time. He looked very upset and was sobbing, his shoulders gently rising and falling. His name was Jake, he told me. I had no time to prepare for what was coming.

"I've wanted to kill myself," he said in a high, out-of-breath voice filled with desperation. "I just want to kill myself. I'm so ashamed," he blurted out. His tears were now spotting his shirt. Everyone had left the gym. Jake and I were mercifully alone with his pain until a custodian suddenly appeared and began unceremoniously folding the dozens and dozens of metal chairs. The thunderclap noise echoed off the gym's block walls and high ceiling, making it nearly impossible to hear. I put my hand gently on Jake's back and ushered him to a more shielded spot in the vestibule of the gym's side entrance. Fortunately, there were two metal chairs there leaning against the wall. I opened them and asked Jake to sit. At least the small space offered us some privacy. I sat down next to him with my arm around his shoulder trying to calm him. His face was flushed and his eyes were rimmed in red.

"I feel so depressed," he told me. "I just can't go on like

this." He was in the seventh grade. My heart was racing. I had been suddenly swept into the life and pain of a young boy that I knew nothing about just a minute earlier. It frightened me how quickly Jake opened up to me, a person he had never met. But he had heard my story and knew I would understand; that I would not tell him to stop saying such things; that I might have some special wisdom to help him persevere. I was honored by his trust but acutely aware that I very much still needed to earn it. I just hoped I could.

Once we were alone, Jake began crying harder and spoke in spurts while trying to catch his breath. "I don't know why I feel like I do," he blurted out. "I just can't live like this anymore. I don't like my life. I can't stop thinking about killing myself," he said in anguish. I began rubbing his back, trying to calm him down as best I could. He was a cute kid with closely cropped brown hair and hazel eyes that seemed to sparkle through his tears. But his suffering was palpable.

"Why are you feeling so sad, Jake, and so desperate?" I asked him softly. "It's hard to see you so upset. Can you tell me what you think is going on?"

Jake turned slowly and stared up at me. Tears were flowing freely down his cheeks. "I don't know why. School, friends, my life. I just feel terrible. I am so ashamed that I want to kill myself." To try to get him talking, I asked about his family and whether he had shared his feelings with his parents. "My mother tries to talk to me," he confided, "but she wants me to see a counselor. I don't want to do that. I'm too ashamed."

I paused and began slowly rubbing his back again. "I think I know why you're ashamed," I said in a low, confidential voice like I was about to share a secret.

"Why?" he asked.

"Because you made a bad choice when you decided to feel like this. That's why you're ashamed," I told him.

Looking right at me, he hesitated, critically processing what I had just told him. After a second or two, he responded with a slight edginess in his voice. "I didn't choose it," he said. "It's not my fault."

"Then what are you ashamed of?" I asked. "Why would you be ashamed of something you didn't do; something you never chose?"

He studied me intently. "What should I do?" he asked.

"Jake, none of what you are feeling is your fault. I could have the same feelings you do, and I wouldn't have chosen them either," I said to assure him. He had stopped crying. "But the feelings you told me about are real and you were very brave and smart to tell me. Let me tell you what I'd like you to do. I'd like you to talk with your mom today when she gets home. She loves you a lot and wants to get you the help you need. You should listen to her. I think if you do and you go see that counselor she mentioned, you'll begin to feel better. Will you do that for me?" I asked.

"OK," he replied, "if you think I should." I could tell I had broken through.

"I really do, Jake. I want your time in middle school to not feel as it does now. I bet the counselor will help."

We both stood as if on cue. He seemed so small for such a grown-up discussion. But at least, I thought, he was brave enough to have it.

"I have to go or I'll be late for my next period," he hurriedly declared.

"Good luck with everything, Jake," I said.

As he started toward the vestibule door, he turned quickly, took a step back and gave me a tight hug. "Thanks for talking with me," he said with relief in his voice. With that, he turned, opened the door and disappeared into the throng of students shuttling down the corridor.

When the door closed, I sat down in the closet-like stillness around me, lost in the emotion of that encounter. Ten minutes earlier, he and I were unknown to each other. Now he had pulled me into his young life, and I felt acutely invested in him. I thought about him all the way home.

I returned to the middle school that night at 7:00 p.m. to give my talk to parents. Turnout at the evening talks for parents was often disappointing. Some of that was due to hectic work and family schedules, but some of it no doubt was the uncomfortable nature of the subject and the fear that other parents might wonder if their son or daughter had "problems." Even today, mental health is still one of those topics adults shy away from discussing.

But this night was different. More than 100 parents attended. As they filed into the gym, singly and in groups of two and three, chatting with aquaintances, a tall woman in her early 40s walked directly toward me. While she extended her hand to shake mine, her demeanor seemed subtlety unfriendly.

"Did you talk to my son this morning?" she asked curtly.

"I may have ma'am. I talked to a lot of kids who wanted to talk with me."

"My son is Jake. Do you remember him?" she asked with a stern gaze.

"Actually, I do. Jake was the last student I spoke to. He was having a real hard time. I tried to comfort him." I braced myself because I had no idea what was coming next but my instincts prepared me to expect a rebuke.

"When Jake came home, he told me that a judge had come to his school this morning and talked about mental illness. He said the two of you later spoke and that you told him that what was bothering him was not his fault."

"I did, ma'am. I encouraged him to talk with you. He said you were encouraging him to see a counselor. That made sense to me." I was expecting she would next tell me to mind my own business. I steeled myself.

Surprisingly, her face softened into a warm smile. "Thanks for talking to Jake," she said. "He just wouldn't listen to me. You know, mothers. But he said you told him that his negative feelings weren't his fault. He said, 'Mom, he was a judge so he must know what he's talking about.' And now he's agreed to see the counselor. I came tonight to thank you." I grabbed her right hand in both of mine and told her she had made my day. The rest of the evening was a blur after that.

I remember giving the principal a note of encouragement I had written that afternoon to give the next day to the boy in the wheelchair, and I remembered all the faces and stories of those courageous kids that I would never see again and never forget.

I wish you were with me on my journey to discovery. You would be impacted, too. You would be just as impatient for change as I am.

PART II

REFLECTIONS AND CHOICES

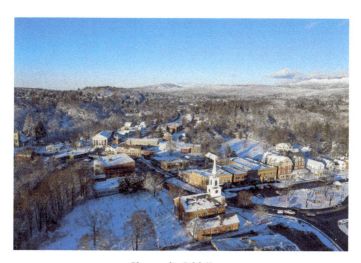

Photo credit: Caleb Kenna

As I look back on the last six years, I readily acknowledge that I don't have the medical or mental health training to offer tested or peer-reviewed insights into all that I have seen and experienced—or the formal training to discern all the cultural forces and societal pressures stressing and shaping the adolescents who have confided in me. But I have been privileged to talk to more kids in these last six years than many who do. They have been my teachers. My empirical knowledge gleaned from thousands of confided conversations with students in almost 300 gyms and auditoriums has deeply affected me. As a trial lawyer and judge for almost four decades, I pride myself on being a good listener and on my ability to understand, discern and communicate what I have heard and seen. From the pain of my family's journey, replete with my mistakes and failings, my son's courage and insights and the confidences shared with me by thousands of adolescents, I believe my impressions have their own independent value and authenticity. I feel a responsibility to share them.

To address what I have seen and learned, I feel certain of three things. First, we need a new and different conversation and vocabulary around mental health to finally remove the stigma that for generations has left too many people ashamed, alone and imperiled. Second, we need to be wise enough and patient enough to "stop the film" to discuss and identify the cultural and societal changes and pressures that are negatively affecting the mental health of America's youth. While mental illness can have many different originating causes—from DNA to adverse childhood experiences to chemical imbalance—I believe most of what I have seen and hugged has its roots in the ever-evolving and complex Petri dish of the 21st century. Finally, we need to lead a movement to create a mental health system in

America that is real, open, accessible and affordable for everyone, especially the young. We are a long way from that now. There is much work to be done.

My travels these past six years have allowed me to go over "the next hill" to the valley beyond to meet and engage in very personal ways with the generation that is coming in our direction. They will one day be leading our country, raising families, populating our professions, running businesses large and small and doing the hard work to make America better. I know firsthand their incredible strengths, and I also know the very real mental health challenges they are enduring. We owe it to them—and ourselves—to listen to what they are telling us, learn from them and then act. Anything less will come at a cost none of us will want.

What has remained with me from my experiences speaking to students and hearing their stories in public and private schools across northern New England is how this current generation of middle school and high school students is stressed, anxious and depressed to a level I don't ever recall seeing or experiencing when I was their age. They are clearly smarter, more open, more worldly wise and less judgmental than any prior generation of Americans, and for that, they have my admiration. But many are experiencing a widening gap between their chronological age and their emotional growth that seemed substantially narrower to nonexistent in my youth. Between 2009 and 2019, one out of three high school students reported persistent feelings of sadness and hopelessness (depression). That represents a 40 percent increase over the previous decade. One out of six high school students reported "making a plan to kill themselves" in the past year. That's a 44 percent increase since 2009. How much longer can we turn away from this reality and pretend it's not our kids, our schools or our community?

Less than half of these kids who are suffering are getting any professional help, and their problems will not just get better on their own or fade away with time.

I have traveled tens of thousands of miles these last several years in every season on main highways and backroads in an effort to start a new and nonjudgmental conversation about mental illness in all its forms and from all its causes to take away the crippling shame and stigma that has existed for generations; a shame and stigma that I bought into for much of my life without much thought. But I was ignorant then. I'm not ignorant now. I was apparently tolerant of intolerance then. Not anymore.

In the course of these last several years, speaking at more than 300 middle schools and high schools in communities large and small, congested and rural, I have hugged or been hugged by several thousand kids who heard my story and then courageously confided their own. I wish you could have been with me on those days. I wish you could have seen their faces and the pain in their eyes. The trust and vulnerability of those kids have touched me deeply and opened me to the daily pressures, traumatic events, incessant technology and ever-rising expectations of parents and the impatient world that are sculpting their lives.

This generation is facing challenges that were better managed, less intrusive and often nonexistent when I was their age. None of them was born before 9/11. Many of them have not enjoyed the simplicity and emotional growth of unstructured after-school play, the gift of unscheduled time, the comfort of undistracted parents at home in the evening, shared family dinners almost every night and the emotional security of a neighborhood that knows their parents and keeps a watchful eye. Today's kids have never experienced a world without social media, the ubiquitous selfie and constant electronic communication. Sadly, many are addicted to a virtual world that is playing an outsized, invisible and incredibly formative role in shaping who they are and how they relate and connect to everyday life.

One night, my wife and I were having dinner at a local restaurant. As we were nearing the end of our meal, a mother, father and their four daughters, who appeared to be between 9 to 14, were shown to a table a short distance from ours. After a few minutes, my wife whispered to me, "Look at that family." When I did, I noticed that all six had their eyes on their phones or tablets. No one was talking. They were all around the same table but they were emotionally and socially alone. Once they gave their orders, they returned to their devices. They remained silent with heads down for the full 15 minutes before our check arrived. They were still looking down when we left. Going out to dinner with my parents and my sister when I was a kid was a big deal. We always talked as a family as we waited for dinner, and I often learned a lot just listening to my parents talking with each other and to friends of theirs who occasionally stopped by our table. Unfortunately, my memorable experiences and their value seem antiquated today. But the growing absence of "being present to others" live and in-person bespeaks a larger problem that I find in a lot of the kids I hug: alone together. Young people are now spending a quarter to a third of their waking hours in the virtual world with no guide or real appreciation for its many inauthentic images and messages. Parents seem unable to control it even when they think they are because they are often too busy traversing the same virtual world, and often at the same time, as their kids. While there can be no doubt that fingertip access to the world has extraordinary value, I'm convinced there is no social or emotional growth on screens, and that social media addiction comes at a cost—not only the depression and anxiety it often causes or exacerbates but also with lost opportunities to create simple yet strengthening memories with family. As far as I was concerned, that family's dinner was a wasted opportunity.

Some days after a long ride home, the stories and suffering of kids I have met and hugged have kept me awake and wondering. I feel a connection to this generation I might never have experienced but for my own failings to see mental illness in my oldest son when he was their age and the painful journey of mistakes and awakening that followed. Those unimaginable years led me to the mental health awareness campaign that has consumed so many of my days and nights and allowed me to enter and be touched by lives I would never have known. My son is proud of my efforts, and I am proud of his courage and perseverance. He has been my teacher on my journey to awareness, too. The stories kids have shared with me, a person they never met and will never likely see again, have left deep imprints that won't fade or wear away. Rather, they have made me more and more impatient for change.

Their trust has caused me to reflect not only upon their suffering but also on how I could have been blind to them and, more importantly, what all of us can do to help them. I don't recall their common afflictions from my youth. If my experiences when I was their age had been comparable to what I've seen these last several years, I'm certain I would have known it. Somehow, somewhere. But I never saw it. Its apparent absence can't be explained away simply by the cultural reluctance to talk about social and emotional health when I was young, although that was no doubt a part of it. The awkwardness and stigma surrounding that topic no doubt kept people ashamed and in denial.

But even making allowances for that cultural camouflage and general ignorance, today's statistics on student mental health are alarming. Stress, anxiety and depression that often change, diminish or even take kids' lives are epidemic among America's youth. Suicide rates for those between the ages of 10 and 24, according to the CDC, increased by 56 percent from 2007 to 2017. That isn't just happening for no apparent reason. During my 12 years of school in a Massachusetts town of 20,000 people, I never heard of any student taking their own life or even trying to. Few students in school today will be able to make that claim. But suicide is not the only disturbing statistic. As that high school principal in Meredith said to me the morning I spoke to his students, "If you haven't been in a high school in the last 10 years, you've never been in a high school." I thought that was hyperbole then but no longer. And he wasn't talking about the building.

Before I began my six-year odyssey promoting mental health awareness, I had never heard of YRBS. I know about it now. The CDC has been making these standardized behavioral survey questionnaires available to school districts across the United States every other year since the early 1990s. Many high schools use them. The survey has dozens of multiple-choice questions exploring numerous topics including alcohol use, sexual practices, dating violence, drug use, bullying and many more. The students completing the survey only identify themselves by sex, age and year in school. In every other way, the students are anonymous. The questions that caught my attention most related principally to depression, suicide and non-lethal self-harm.

In some geographic regions in New Hampshire, upwards of 45 percent of high school girls identified themselves as depressed, and one in four students said they had "seriously considered" taking their own life during the past 12 months. An alarming percentage of those acknowledged "making plans" to kill themselves in that same time frame. A measurable percent of students actually tried to end their own lives during the previous year. Nationally that number stands at about seven percent. In 2019, the number was 11 percent among high school girls. In a high school of a thousand students evenly divided by sex, that percentage translates to 55 girls. That was not my world growing up. In many schools, one in five students or more is engaging in non-lethal self-harm. Cutting is the most common. I still remember the two middle-school girls who asked me after my talk if I knew what cutting was. When I said I did, I asked if they knew kids in their school who were cutting. They looked at each other quickly before pushing up their sleeves to reveal their cut arms. They were in the eighth grade. We shared a group hug and I asked them if they were getting help. Thankfully they were, but many aren't.

The YRBS numbers for mental health in New Hampshire sadly track a lot of the national averages. I was stunned when I first read them. But I was even more stunned that they weren't front-page news or even commonly discussed. I only knew of them because I was alerted to their existence by a high school principal who assumed I had seen them. I couldn't understand why parents weren't reacting with alarm. It was unimaginable to me. But no longer. In my many conversations with school administrators, I learned that the survey results are rarely shared directly with parents. Some told me the results went to central school administration and often to the local school boards. Most acknowledged that nothing was sent home. In New Hampshire, the Department of Education publishes the gross survey numbers for the state as well as the numbers averaged by geographic region. But the website does not share the results for individual schools. I doubt most parents are even aware those numbers are on the website. If 45 percent of high school girls had leukemia or diabetes or Covid-19, it would be a front-page, above-the-fold story and declared a public health emergency. Somehow, alarming depression and suicide ideation numbers remain below the radar.

One day, a senior education official shared the only answer that made sense, as sad as it was. "If we tell the parents [about the YRBS numbers], they will blame us," she told me. From my travels, I came to the view that schools are not the problem and, in fact, are doing more than almost anyone else to address the mental health challenges in their classrooms and hallways. School counselors are on the front lines and often in need of reinforcements. I didn't understand how schools could be blamed or should feel defensive. But oddly, that is the case. Increasingly, schools today are perceived as the "dry cleaners" for America's youth. They are expected to address all manner of issues, mental health included, that they didn't cause and don't get to go home with when the bell rings. They have been burdened with a near-impossible task. They need our help, especially when it comes to mental health. Many schools now have trained counselors to deal with the numerous challenges and issues kids present, but most often their attention is focused on dealing with the ever-rising stress, anxiety and depression among students. In spring 2019, in support of my travels on mental health, Dartmouth Health held a youth summit to let high school students discuss the challenges their generation is confronting. The four-member student teams from 63 public high schools across New Hampshire met in Concord on two consecutive days. The forum discussions were student-led and informal. They focused on topics from gender to race to bullying to mental health. Experts were there to answer questions, but not to direct discussion. The students offered several recommendations on day two.

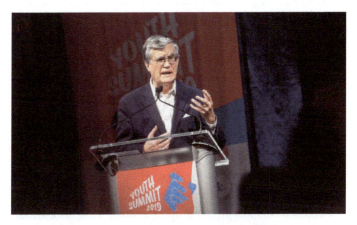

In spring 2019, in support of John's travels on mental health, Dartmouth Health held a youth summit to let high school students discuss the challenges their generation is confronting. (Photo credit: Kata Sasvari)

One was a need for "more counselors and more specialized counselors in [their] schools." The students were speaking for their generation. I couldn't have imagined a consensus recommendation remotely close to that from my high school class of baby boomers. But my last six years of speaking, listening, hugging and learning have helped me add real context to their plea and underscore its urgency. I see the need. I support their call for help. We need to listen to these kids. They are speaking to us. Unfortunately, I'm not sure we're listening.

This generation is being raised in a Petri dish unlike any prior generation. The barrier between night and day has eroded as has the barrier between home and work and home and school. A tough day at school can now follow you home. You can now be bullied in the quiet of your bedroom at any hour. You can be defamed or maligned before all your classmates at the click of a mouse, night or day. You can make a teenage mistake online that will follow you forever. None of that is good for mental and emotional health. The notion of being "safe at home" no longer applies. The virtual world has removed walls and social boundaries. Sometimes that happens to a great advantage, but not always. A mother recently told me that she found her 10th-grade daughter asleep on her own bed in her own room, fully clothed at 1:30 a.m. with her laptop open on her stomach and two classmates watching her sleep. The mother opined that this generation seems afraid to be alone. I wondered why? Ironically, even when kids are constantly "connected" online, they are often still alone.

Today's kids are growing up in a world of school shootings, foreign and domestic terrorism, unparalleled political divisiveness, 24/7 news and constant image-centric social media. They are over-stressed, over-supervised, over-organized, over-competing and over-anxious. One high school student, a varsity co-captain of his school's hockey team, told me that every day he goes to school he perceives and experiences a low but constant level of anxiety throughout his building and among his classmates. His friends, he confided, are on their iPhones six or seven hours a day outside of school. Although he fights it, he feels pressure to portray an unrealistic version of himself on social media to please his friends and "followers." Sometimes, the smiling person on the screen surrounded by the "cool kids" is not who he is or how he feels. But the virtual world makes unrelenting demands. He is not alone. There are more iPhones on after midnight than most parents want to admit. Maybe theirs are, too.

Parents, acting with the best of intentions, have too often been reluctant to let this generation grow through the unchaperoned, sometimes trying, trial-and-error experiences of childhood. Kids are missing out on the childhood I remember, and I believe are losing out on the social/emotional growth it gave me. "Be home for dinner" during school nights or "Be home when the streetlights come on" during the endless days of summer vacation have become almost extinct.

In my childhood, I was out playing with my friends almost every afternoon and all weekend. I learned independence and self-reliance. I learned to mediate my disputes and settle differences. We made up our own games with our own rules. We were pretty creative. Most kids I knew never played organized sports before high school, but most were playing sports or games of some kind at the playground, the town common or in someone's driveway or backyard. Organized sports for young people, other than Little League, were almost nonexistent. Adults were available, if you needed them, but were largely invisible. They were not organizing us. Play, so essential in my youth and to my development and self-discovery, is now seen too often as time wasted when kids "should be learning a skill," "practicing something" or "doing homework." Even recess has fallen into disfavor. Recess was something my generation looked forward to in grade school.

Commenting on the death of recess in the lives of children, Professor Peter Gray of Boston College noted in his book *Free to Learn*: "When I was an elementary school student in the 1950s, we had half-hour recesses each morning and afternoon, and we were free to do whatever we wished, even leave the school grounds." I can relate. I went home each day for lunch to meet my mother (who came home from work just for lunch) during our one-hour break. I walked home and back by myself. Today, that would be considered too much time and likely too dangerous. This reflection should not be seen as a halcyon reference to "the good old days" but rather as a recognition that a generation ago kids were given space and time to grow and mature on the road to self-reliance.

I fear that kids growing up today are on too tight a leash, are too over-structured and too dependent on adult supervision. We are unwittingly shortening and short-changing childhood. That comes with consequences. I have hugged some of them. Creativity, imagination and resilience are suffering. So is self-confidence. Adolescents are strapped to their iPhones, and parents too often call them multiple times a day to check in. Parents are often driven by fear for their child's safety, although studies show that those fears are overblown. Letting your children head out on their bicycles to roam the neighborhood and beyond, as my generation did every summer day, seems too risky now for many parents. Fences come with consequences.

In recent years, I've rarely seen kids "out playing." As Professor Gray perceptively observed, "It used to be that you could walk through any neighborhood in America, after school or on weekends, or during the summer, and see children playing outside without adult supervision. Now if you see them outside at all, they are likely to be wearing uniforms and following the directions of adult coaches, while their parents look on and dutifully cheer their every move." Today, I fear that if you suggested to some kids that they head outside to play, they might ask, "Play what?" or "Is that an 'app?'"

When one of my granddaughters was just five, she was playing on a soccer team with a volunteer coach. They played a "rigorous" three-game schedule. My wife and I drove to Connecticut to be at her last game. The kids ran around the field, kicking the ball. Sometimes the ball was airborne and bouncing off kids in all directions. The coaches yelled instructions. Our granddaughter never seemed to get within 30 feet of the ball. She often seemed to be running in the opposite direction. During the game, I turned to my wife and said, "Lily is either the best defensive soccer player in the world, or she is afraid she might get kicked in the shins." But at the end of the game, every player on Lily's team, all decked out in their color-coordinated uniforms, got what looked like a gold medal the size of your fist strung over their necks on a beautiful, multi-colored ribbon. Lily hung it on the doorknob of her bedroom when she got home. As sweet as it was, I wondered what lessons she had learned.

Schools have become caught up in it, too. When my wife was teaching in her late 40s, she was aghast to see four first-place prizes awarded at the end-of-year grade school competitions. Apparently, she learned, second, third and fourth place were seen as too deflating to acknowledge. In my life experience, and yours I'll bet, not everyone gets a gold medal and not everyone has earned one. Adolescents need to learn from disappointment as well as success. It will definitely be a part of their lives, and they need to be equipped for the inevitable when it comes. Unfortunately, many aren't. That's on us.

One day, I spoke to a star high school athlete and asked if he thought too many parents were living vicariously through their children. With no hesitation, he replied, "100 percent." It all comes at a price. Stress ratchets up.

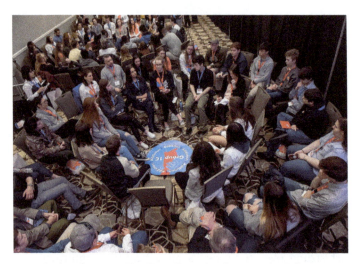

Students from across New Hampshire gathered in Concord, NH, for the two-day Youth Summit hosted by New Hampshire's Dartmouth Health. (Photo credit: Kuta Sasvari)

Too many kids I have talked with have told me of the pressure they feel to be successful, get good grades, make the team. I will always remember the eighth-grader who told me she "freaked out" if she didn't get a 100 on every test. Failure is feared at all levels.

Some years ago, when I was a law school dean, famed lawyer and former Solicitor General of the United States Ted Olson told our graduates that he "learned more from his failures than his successes." Failure had obviously not proven fatal for him nor will it for today's youth. But fear of failure is crippling. I see it almost every time I speak at schools. Too many kids are rushing to catch the train of success. One high school athlete told me that he didn't know where the train was headed or who laid the tracks, but he knew he had to be on it and to move as far forward in the train as he could once he caught it. That was not my high school mandate. I never felt that pressure at that level, ever. Sadly, many kids feel that pressure every day now.

Many of the students I have spoken with after my remarks often seem distraught over academic expectations. Everyone is competing in a constant march to recognition and achievement. Outcome fever is a common virus. Parents are keeping score and some are posting—and bragging—about it online. Making it to the first car on the train is seen as imperative for many of these students, but getting to the front seats of the first car seems equally important. Increasingly, students from a young age are treated as "small adults in waiting": waiting to become a lawyer, a doctor, an engineer or a Division I college athlete. No time can be wasted on self-discovery or just "hanging out." Downtime is wasted time apparently. Internships and "the right summer job" are often sought after by high school students to enhance resumes for college. But even success is often not sufficiently satisfying. One young man told me that even when his classmates get into their "dream school" for college, they don't seem that happy. They need to be off to the next accomplishment and can't take the time to enjoy the good news.

In a neighboring town around graduation a year or so ago, my wife and I noticed a sign in a front yard of a very upscale home declaring the owners to be "PROUD PARENTS" of a local high school graduate. About two weeks later, the sign was down and replaced with one of the college their son or daughter would be attending, announcing he/she would be a member of the class of 2024. I doubt their child put the sign up. A few weeks later, we drove by another elegant home sitting on a lot with cascading hills descending down to the street. Prominently displayed on one of those embankments was a carefully spray-painted four-foot "S" on specially cut grass in Syracuse University colors. We were not sure what to make of that. In the world I came from, where I got into college was not of billboard importance. The people who wanted to know where I was going beyond my circle of friends was a fairly small group. My mother and father would never have allowed me to spray paint our front lawn purple for Holy Cross—or any other color—but neither I nor they would have ever thought to do it. Something has changed. Our kids are affected by it.

One day, when I was leaving yet another auditorium through a side exit, I encountered a student waiting to talk with me in the near-empty hallway. "The line was pretty long in there," she said. "I thought I might be able to catch you out here before you left." She was a junior, she told me. She had a round face, shoulder-length hair and wore an unhappy frown.

"Happy to talk with you," I told her. "You waited a long time. Is this a good place to talk?" I asked.

She looked so forlorn. "This is fine," she said without any inflection. She then began her disclosure to a perfect stranger. "I'm in all Advanced Placement classes here," she started, then paused.

In an effort to lighten her mood, I said, "There should be a law against people like you. No one should be allowed to be that smart." My comment only drew a meek smile.

"It's not that good," she replied, "I study every night until 11:30. I have no life." She then looked down. That had not been my junior year in high school. I'm not sure how many Advance Placement courses there were in my school, but I wasn't in any if they existed.

"Why are you doing that?" I asked her.

She looked up. "To please my parents."

"I don't know your parents," I said, "but I am sure they

love you very much and wouldn't want you feeling like you do. Have you talked to them and told them what you told me?" I asked softly.

"No," she replied.

"Well, I think you should," I told her. "I'm certain it would make you feel better." She never committed to doing it but moved forward to hug me, and then she was off. She had waited almost 40 minutes to see me after I had spoken. She just needed to tell someone. I hope she talked to her parents, but I have my doubts. Maybe a sign will go up in her front yard when she graduates, but I know she won't be the one requesting it.

Too many kids are constantly in motion. A mother of four adolescents confided in me one day that she felt like the "CEO of her kids' color-coded calendars." One of her sons confirmed to me that he had almost no free time. Every hour of his high school life was booked. When I asked him how many of his friends got eight hours of sleep a night, he laughed. "Nobody does that," he said. "Most nights I only get five or six hours myself." In fact, according to the CDC, almost 80 percent of adolescents go on less than eight hours of sleep. And before they head out the door to school each morning, more than 65 percent have no breakfast one or more days a week. Tired and hungry are not usually considered the stepping-stones to success, but they are often associated with depression and anxiety. When I told him that most of my high school weekends were free to do whatever I wanted, he quipped, "I can't relate to that." He longingly followed up, "I can't imagine what that would be like." In short, he couldn't imagine my childhood. I couldn't imagine his, either. A classmate of his, also a smart, successful varsity athlete, confessed to me that he felt like he didn't really have a childhood.

Kids have lamented to me that they are not free to make mistakes. "You only really learn by making mistakes," one young man told me, "but parents won't let us." More and more parents, it seems, are plowing the roads, smoothing out the bumps and filling in the potholes for their children. Adversity and struggle are increasingly to be avoided at all costs. Like most people my age, I learned a lot from mine. While I have no doubt that parents are coming from a good place, their protective envelope is unwittingly retarding social and emotional growth in their kids.

On one of my visits to a private school in New Hampshire, I spoke to an assembly of several hundred students in grades six through 12. The auditorium was full. The kids in the front few rows looked so young to me. I was just hoping my talk could keep everyone's attention and span the age range from 11 to 18. It seemed a daunting task. It was pin-drop quiet as I talked. When I finished, the first kids standing and applauding were those young faces in the front rows—the very faces I thought were way too young to understand my impatience for change, in fact, shared my impatience. Soon the whole room was standing. A part of me quietly hopes every time I speak, as uncomfortable as it would be, that my remarks fall flat and that kids look perplexed. That never happens. The kids understand. They know. They live it.

On my way out of the auditorium that morning, I struck up a conversation with the dean of students. I asked how technology was handled at their school. "We have a new problem," he told me. "We don't allow students to use their iPhones in class, but now parents are texting their kids during class, and they want a prompt reply. It's hard to have rules when the kids comply and the parents don't," he said in resigned frustration.

As he was walking me toward my car, I asked him how parents were when it came to academic success. "Everyone has high expectations here," he told me. "Recently, we had parent/teacher night after a marking period. The parents of a sixth-grader went to see their son's teacher to complain." Apparently, they had his report card and put it down on the teacher's desk. "These are not our son's grades," the mother said. When the teacher confirmed that they were her son's grades, her husband jumped in.

"With the money we're paying to send him here, we can't accept those grades." As I drove home that day, I thought I had probably hugged that kid many times in many places. I could hear the whistle of the train he would be running to catch—and he was only a sixth-grader. I reflected that when I was his age, I was still trying to improve my penmanship, hoping my teacher would allow me to continue to write with my left hand.

Many parents and grandparents, like I was, are still caught up in yesterday's thinking when it comes to mental illness. They learned or avoided just as I had. Many fear the very label of mental illness and believe it's hopeless if acknowledged. They worry that their kids might be "coded" or penalized or ostracized in some way if they are seen as having a mental health challenge. They fear that any record of it might hurt their college admission or employment prospects. Still others fear that acknowledging it in their child implicates them in some unflattering way. Many in their generations learned that mental illness was rare, a weakness, a character flaw or even an excuse. Too many of us have bought into the "code of silence" and the culture that created it.

Some students have shared with me that their parents don't "believe" in mental illness or just instruct them to "get over it" or assure them that they "will grow out of whatever is bothering them." The world still has too many excuses for the mental health conditions it sees or avoids seeing for what they are. Many school counselors have told me that while some parents are relieved to discuss their child's mental health when they reach out to them, many others are not open to talking about it. I likely would have been one of those disbelieving parents, so I am not maligning or judging them. But I know now from tragic personal experience and thousands of conversations with middle school and high school students that ignorance is not our friend when it comes to mental illness. It never has been.

Although I have never spoken to grade-school kids, I would from time to time speak to teachers and staff at grade schools. I will never forget my first experience there. It was the end of the day, and I was walking down a long, brightly colored corridor with the principal on our way to the lunchroom where folks were assembling. There were still a few children hurriedly grabbing things from their lockers along our route in their mad dash to catch the school bus or to meet a waiting parent. I was suddenly flooded with my own memories of those long-ago days of total innocence. As we were walking, I said casually to the principal, "Thanks for the opportunity you are giving me today but I'm sure you don't see mental health issues here." Her brow suddenly furrowed. She gently touched my right forearm and brought us both to a stop.

"I wish that was true," she said regretfully. "We have a third-grade girl in a mental health hospital and a second-grade boy who finally convinced enough of us that he was serious when he told us he was going to kill himself." Those were not my memories of grade school but it was her reality and the kids' reality. I was shaken by what she told me and felt almost overwhelmed by what I hadn't realized; by what I had never seen. In the years to follow, the shock I felt that afternoon was replaced with impatience. The candor of the kids changed me.

I ask almost every upset student who approaches me in confidence, after I share my family's story, if they are getting help anywhere. More than half are not. That's consistent with national statistics. Some don't think their family can afford it, some are afraid, some say their parents don't think they need it, some don't believe their pain can be addressed, some are embarrassed, some are describing the conditions of friends or siblings they worry about and some blame themselves for their own suffering.

As the years passed and I spoke with more and more kids about their challenges and struggles, I invariably wondered as I reflected on my ride home if their parents saw and knew what I was seeing and hearing or, at least, perceived it the same way if they did. I knew the parents of the kids who were brave enough to open up to me had daily lives and pressures as unfamiliar to me as those confronting and sometimes disabling their children. The parents' days were lived at an ever-accelerating speed with blurred boundaries between home and work and fueled by career and cultural demands to compete and achieve. Many parents, whatever their station, find themselves as tethered to technology as their own kids, just not as proficient. They have more demands on their private space and less free time than my parents ever had—than I have had, too—and they believe that their kids have to know more and do more than they had known or done to compete and win in a global world. I don't doubt that their intentions are pure or that they want more for their kids than they had themselves. That's the hope of every American generation. But I wonder whether this generation is paying too high a price. I also wonder if we are all too busy to notice or reflect on what I have been seeing and hugging. But maybe I had been too busy, too.

The hardest group for me to reach on my mental health awareness campaign has been parents, and it's not for lack of trying. Students are a captive audience but parents don't assemble easily. I appreciate how hard it is for them to come out for an evening event, especially during the week, so I am not unsympathetic. They no doubt have a lot of competing interests and responsibilities and going to an evening talk about mental health likely doesn't jump to the top of their "to-do" list. But in my many talks with school principals, I've learned that parents rarely assemble in large numbers at schools these days for any reason other than sports. But I always try to attract them.

I spoke one morning at a small, combined middle and high school in New Hampshire. My talk went well, and the students lined up to talk. Before I left, I met with the principal and the head counselor. I asked them if I could return at some point for an evening event with parents. They immediately lowered my expectations. "Don't get me wrong and please don't take it personally," the principal said, "because mental health issues are common here, but parents just won't come out to hear you." Feeling like she owed me an explanation, the principal continued. "This past September, after we had been in session less than a month, I personally invited all the parents to come here one evening to meet their kids' teachers and say hello to our administrative staff. I thought I should provide some food, so I ordered 10 large pizzas. When the night was over, nine boxes remained untouched," she said with an edge of sadness in her voice. "I was very disappointed." Needless to say, I never returned to speak, but I couldn't shake the sorry image of a pyramid of unopened pizza boxes and what they represented. I just hoped the kids I spoke with one-on-one that day had parents who knew about their suffering and were addressing it.

Another evening, having spoken that morning to students at a large high school in a very upscale town, I came back to speak to parents. The principal had sent a personal email several weeks earlier to the entire school community describing my talk and underscoring its importance. The turnout was underwhelming. The principal was apologetic, but not surprised. "A few nights ago, we had to turn parents away," he told me. "The basketball team had a playoff game here. This place was mobbed." I couldn't help but wonder whether any of those players was dealing with depression or anxiety or both. My travels had shown me that athletes weren't immune. I know because I have hugged them. In my experience, it seems sometimes harder for high school athletes to discuss their mental health struggles with their parents. I still remember a football lineman who spoke to me privately after one of my talks. He shared his growing depression and anxiety with me.

"Have you talked to your parents about this?" I asked him.

"I could never tell my parents," he replied.

"If you hurt your knee and weren't able to play in Saturday's game, would you tell them that?" I asked.

"Sure," he said. "But mental health is different." He had obviously learned the lessons previous generations had handed down. Thankfully, he agreed to talk for the first time to a counselor at the school. Unfortunately, he is not alone in his reluctance. That's on all of us, too.

ONE DAY, I spoke to 1,600 students in four assemblies. More than 125 kids waited to speak to me when my remarks concluded. Hugs were plentiful. That evening, I returned to speak to parents. Only 42 attended, and they represented fewer than 42 students. The principal seemed quite surprised. Sadly, based on my previous experiences, I wasn't. If it had been an evening devoted to success and not struggles, I suspect that many more parents would have attended.

In so many of my confided conversations with students, they shared their feelings and angst with me about the stress brought on by everyday life and seemed almost fearful of its demands and expectations. Some were chasing academic rabbits to please their parents or to get into their "dream school" (whether it was really their dream or not), some were mostly focused on sports for the elusive scholarship and almost all were trying to maintain their status or improve it on social media while some were being made to feel less valued and less included on its screens. I had the sense from many of the kids I hugged that they were afraid to disappoint and even more afraid to fail, however they defined that. In one very competitive upscale New Hampshire high school, it was reported in the media that some students, when learning about a possible surprise quiz later in the day, would go to the nurse and ask to be released from school. Parents were often called, and the students would be driven home. I hated quizzes as much as they did, but ducking out was never an option for me, and my parents would not have seen it as an option either.

The virtual world is the "new neighborhood" for this generation. It's a place to make "friends," show off your "likes," share your videos and post your "isn't my life perfect" selfies to gain acceptance and followers. But it's missing what kids need and what most of us grew up with—a sense of belonging and a feeling that we mattered to others as we explored who we were and might become. We felt protected.

Despite its wonders, the "new neighborhood" can become a driver of anxiety, self-doubt, unrelenting pressure and depression. The virtual world never stops, never takes a break nor allows kids to take one. It's awake and running 24/7 and its addictive pull comes with consequences. I remember a high school principal told me that one day when he stepped into his outer office, he saw a sophomore girl standing by the counter crying hysterically. He went to her aid immediately. "Young lady," he said with some urgency in his voice, "What's wrong? What's happened?" It ended up that she had been brought to her visibly distraught state because her close friend, a student in the very same high school, had not texted her back after an hour. Time and immediacy have new meaning and expectations for this generation, but their new demands come at a real cost to many kids. Just ask the ones who are sleeping with their iPhones.

It's easy to wax poetic about earlier and simpler times. Every generation believes their youth was better than that of the generations that followed. I fully understand that. But even making allowance for that nostalgic haze, this generation of kids is clearly moving at a pace and under a pressure and bombardment unfamiliar to prior generations. They are constantly multi-tasking to stay ahead, and many excel at it. I admire them, but I have hugged and comforted the downside of this new age in too many school gyms and auditoriums not to realize that everything comes at a price. Stress, anxiety and depression are clearly on the rise. Dramatic increases in youth suicide should be telling us something. They are the canary in the coal mine.

Ironically, this generation is both more connected and more socially isolated than any that preceded it. Norms and expectations for these kids have changed. Childhood is shorter not because it should be but because the luxury of time is less generous. Achievement and accomplishment impatiently await while nurturing is compressed. I am of the firm belief that if nothing changes—if we don't hit the pause button in our communities long enough to openly discuss what I have seen, heard and hugged, and address it—then nothing will change. That would be a tragic mistake.

ONE THING that has become painfully obvious to me these last several years through my conversations with thousands of kids and countless adults is that we don't have a mental health system in America. We never have, really. It's hard to justify since tens of millions of adults will experience a mental health challenge in their lifetimes and one in five adolescents will, too. Those numbers far exceed the totals for all cancers, diabetes, dementia, HIV and ALS combined. As forward-thinking and proactive as we have been on research, treatment and coverage for illnesses and conditions that affect far fewer people than mental illness, a good thing to be sure, we have always fallen short on mental health. Few people are willing to advocate for change for fear their secret or their family's story might be exposed. Stigma and shame are still very real. Much of it derives from fear, ignorance and false pride.

Science and treatment protocols have advanced for mental and emotional health, but access remains a huge and stubborn hurdle. We have too few people entering the field of mental health, and we are doing little to incentivize those career choices. We have only 28,000 psychiatrists practicing in America today. In a nation of more than 330 million people, we are woefully understaffed, and a lot of critical positions below the level of psychiatrist are going unfilled. We need more psychologists, clinical social workers, psychiatric registered nurses, psychiatric nurse practitioners and mental health counselors. All of these shortages exist for a reason and all of them could be eliminated if we create, underwrite and incentivize a real mental health system in our country.

Mental health is still seen by too many people as somehow different from every other physical illness. Even now. To some, it is seen as a choice, a weakness, a lack of rectitude or even an excuse. "Why are you depressed with all your advantages?" or "Just snap out of it!" are refrains we still hear or silently think. Thoughts and questions like these do not exist with cancer, diabetes, ALS and a host of other physical illnesses. No one would ever say, "How can you have cancer with all of your advantages?" or "Why don't you just snap out of it?" if you are suffering from diabetes. That is because we fully accept that cancer and diabetes are health problems and not choices. Sadly, we're still not there with mental illness.

We now know that mental health is entitled to "parity" under the Affordable Care Act, but we also know that is usually honored in the breach. Not only do some insurers push back or seek to cap visits, but mental health providers are often reimbursed at lower rates than many other providers treating better understood physical illnesses. Just the fact that it took generations to achieve insurance "parity" is a clear indication that mental health is seen differently. We don't need to assert that treatment for cancer, heart disease, bad backs and bad knees are entitled to "parity." They are just covered under your health policy. Mental health should be treated with the same respect as every other physical illness. It isn't. If only mental illness could be diagnosed by a blood test, X-ray or MRI, attitudes might change. But it can't and won't. But it is nonetheless very real, very common and very often treatable.

Cancer was once in the shadows during my lifetime, too. My mother used to whisper the word, and many adults wouldn't even do that. "He or she had the c-word," they would solemnly confide in hushed tones. As a child, I wondered why cancer was shrouded in secrecy and shame. Maybe, I thought, if you talked about it out loud you might contract it. Those afflicted never mentioned it to their neighbors, their co-workers or their extended family until it became absolutely necessary. That seems foolish now, but it didn't for generations. It was the norm. In my childhood, I never heard an adult, other than Hugh Hefner of *Playboy* magazine, say the word "breast" in public. Now we say breast cancer and look at the lives that change has saved.

It wasn't that long ago, driven by our general ignorance and fear, that those suffering with the AIDS virus were often declared to be bad people. They were unceremoniously ostracized and stigmatized. But everything began to change when we learned that innocent children could be born with the virus and NBA legend Magic Johnson had to step away as a player in 1991 because he had HIV. Everyone loved Magic. Now there is a "cocktail" of medications, and HIV patients have a very different horizon and are perceived so differently by the broader society. People talk about it openly now without judgment or stigma, as they should, and support those with this illness.

Compared to the social acceptance, striking medical advancements and defined paths for access to treatment for cancer and HIV, mental illness has only inched forward. We don't have the personnel, the facilities, the research dollars, the needed integrated delivery system, the insurance coverage, the appropriate reimbursement rates for providers, the necessary federal and state funding and the appropriate compensation for mental health providers. As a result of these deficiencies, we are turning away from the mental health needs of tens of millions of people who are suffering.

The anemic nature of our mental health system has become painfully obvious during Covid-19. In our state on Valentine's Day 2021, 51 kids and adolescents suffering acute mental health distress were taken to community hospital emergency rooms. Unfortunately, those hospitals were not equipped to provide acute mental health treatment, and kids were kept for days waiting for appropriate beds or treatment to open elsewhere. Boarding is a national problem, and we need state and federal solutions.

While we certainly have some highly talented and dedicated people in mental health and a proven track record that treatment works, we don't have a system. Dr. Will Torrey, the interim department chair of psychiatry at Dartmouth's Geisel School of Medicine and a Harvard Medical School graduate, confirmed it at a November 2019 public forum. When asked how he would rate America's mental health system, his response was to the point. "The way we treat breast cancer today, not 30 years ago, is pretty close to a 10 on a 10-point scale," he told the audience. "We have very good protocols and excellent results. By contrast, mental health is a one or two on that same 10-point scale."

Dr. Benjamin Druss, who holds the Rosalynn Carter Chair in Mental Health in the Department of Health Policy and Management at Emory University and is a nationally recognized expert on access, quality and outcomes of care for those with serious mental illness, was even more sanguine during a recent conversation I had with him. "Calling the mental health system a system is a misnomer," he said. "It's a fragmented patchwork of pieces, and nobody is coordinating the pieces." He went on to describe the state of mental health services in America as "completely and unevenly broken."

For generations, the mentally ill were "out of sight, out of mind." We locked people away in scary, spartan and cruel confines of "lunatic asylums" and "nut houses" where they essentially died twice: the day they were admitted and the day they were buried. They were often chained, isolated, drugged and "shocked" against their will. Lobotomies were not uncommon. Even those suffering from Down syndrome were sent away to "special schools." We knew a family in my childhood that sent their son away. Maybe they had to, but the few times I saw him after church, he seemed kind, devoted and loving to his parents. I always wondered how he felt living away. I couldn't imagine. Today, most Down syndrome children are more visible, more accepted and more mainstreamed. That is a positive development for all of us, especially for them.

Mental illness remains a poor second cousin to virtually every physical illness. It has always been that way. Although some progress has definitely happened over the last 70 years, it remains woefully inadequate. Our checkered history on mental illness includes the perception that those suffering were "possessed," morally deficient, intellectually inferior or of weak character. Mental illness in its many forms and degrees was too often seen as a hopeless affliction. The language we used to describe those who were suffering ranged from insensitive ("mentally retarded") to cruel ("crazy").

Beginning in the mid-1940s with the creation of the National Institute of Mental Health and the allocation of federal funds for mental health research, the development of antipsychotic drugs and enhanced therapy in the 1950s and the signing of The Community Mental Health Act of 1963, the era of deinstitutionalization arrived in earnest. Those "captive" in large and often understaffed and poorly run state psychiatric hospitals were released to their communities where it was believed they could get more effective care from community mental health centers and residential community homes.

During the 1960s and 1970s, hundreds of thousands of previously institutionalized patients were discharged to community treatment, and many state-run facilities were closed or dramatically scaled back. It wasn't a perfect solution but it held promise and demonstrated a more nuanced understanding of mental illness. After 1963, the only people who could be committed to state psychiatric hospitals were those who were an imminent threat to themselves or others. While perhaps well-intentioned, in order to reduce the institutionalized population, Paul Gionfriddo, the president and CEO of Mental Health America, said it had the unintended effect "of making mental health a public safety problem and not the public health problem it actually is." Despite the promise of community mental health centers, the needed level of federal and state funding, principally through Medicaid, never really materialized. As a result, much of the financial burden was shifted to families that were ill-prepared to accept it. And community mental health centers, despite their best efforts, were unable to meet community needs.

In my travels these last six years, I have spoken with many parents after my talks, and sometimes they reach out by phone or email independently. Many have told me about their own children and their Herculean and frustrating efforts to find mental health treatment for them. Sadly, it is a recurring theme. One mother told me about her 14-year-old son who was quite obviously suffering. "I am sure he can be helped," I told her. "Have you made an appointment to have him seen?" She gave me an exhausted half smile.

"I used all my contacts," she said, "but his appointment is four months from now." If her son had broken his hip in their driveway playing basketball, she could have called 911 and they would have sent an ambulance to her house to transport him to the emergency room, and his treatment would be covered by insurance. If your teenager has a chronic mental health problem, who do you call, when can they be seen and what will it cost?

In the course of one three-week span, I received two phone calls soliciting my help. One father had to put his 15-year-old son in residential treatment for the sudden onset of acute mental health problems. It was costing him $1,400 a day. "I feel fortunate that I was able to take out a second mortgage," he told me. "But I don't know how long I will be able to keep him where he is." The second call came from a mother who had her teenager in residential care in Connecticut. She was able to convince her insurance company to let him remain for two weeks but the third week was offloaded on her. She had to pay $2,000 a day. Who can afford health care for children at those prices? How can we justify leaving parents and kids adrift like that? How much longer will the rest of us tolerate that? Sadly, the way we have ignored the needs of the mentally ill, at all levels, is completely immoral.

One morning after I spoke to a group of business professionals, one of the women in the group asked if she could walk me out. The second the elevator doors closed, she began crying. "My son," she said through her sobs, "is going to kill himself when he gets to college next month. He is in a bad way."

"Are you seeing anyone for treatment?" I quickly asked.

"It will be six months before he can get in," she told me barely able to catch her breath.

"We're not going to accept that," I told her. "Let me call someone today at Dartmouth Health." Her son was seen just a few days later. I feared to think what might have happened if she hadn't been brave enough to share her pain and her son's illness, and I hadn't been fortunate enough to work for a premier hospital (itself over-extended in meeting the needs of all those in search of mental health treatment). At present, we just don't have capacity for mental health services in the United States. In fact, we never have. As Dr. Druss told me, "If you're well off, live on the coasts and can afford private pay, you'll find help. If not, it will not be easy to find treatment." According to Dr. Druss, "Most psychiatrists in private practice don't take insurance and of those that do almost no one accepts Medicaid, which is the first line of defense available to poor people." Even when commercial insurance is accepted by a psychiatrist, the reimbursement rates are lower than the reimbursement rates for procedure-based medical care (orthopedics, OB-GYN, neurology, etc.).

Dr. Druss confirmed what I have seen and experienced in my travels and talks. "Stigma still keeps a lot of people away from care," he told me. He also underscored what I have learned these last six years during my many school visits. "School-based mental health services are important," he told me. Those are the very services the students at the Dartmouth Health Summit wanted to see expanded.

We also need an integrated delivery network of pediatricians, family practitioners, internists and mental health professionals. All should be seen in the same silo. According to Dr. Druss, we need to expand mental health services in primary care settings. "We could then diagnose and treat simple issues sooner and refer out the more complex." When that happens, Paul Gionfriddo believes that our health system at the primary and pediatric care level should adopt universal mental health screenings. "That way," he said, "we can focus early on clinical symptoms of mental illness and not wait until stage four as has too often been the case with mental health." At the end of the day, for meaningful and lasting change in the delivery of mental health services, it seems essential that we design a health system that finally integrates physical health, mental health and public health. The rising tide will lift all boats and allow mental health, at last, to be seen and treated for what it is: a health issue. As Dr. Torrey has said, "We need a comprehensive, population-focused health system to identify and address mental health in the United States."

But it will not be easy to build or it would have been built by now. As Dr. Torrey told me, "Discrimination against people with psychiatric illness deeply pervades our society. Getting access to services and treatments that are evidence-based and shown to work is exceedingly hard to do."

After six years of immersion in the mental health challenges of students, listening to their stories and witnessing their pain trying to be understood, trying to gain their footing, and learning of their difficulty in finding treatment and a way forward, it is hard not to conclude that we are failing this generation and their families. Hugging a child who has tried to kill themselves or plans to would change the mind of the worst cynic. I have had that experience many times, and I have no answer, only growing impatience.

I know we can do better than accept a health care system that serves and financially supports what can be physically seen, X-rayed and scanned but woefully neglects the needs of millions of people—some quite young—just as much at risk with conditions not visible but often destructive and debilitating. Those affected are just as deserving of treatment and respect. Sadly, treatment exists that can restore lives and futures but the pathways and needed insurance infrastructure to secure it are too often unbuilt, unfinished, unmarked and unfunded. If we build it, they will come.

Nothing will likely change until we normalize and de-stigmatize mental illness and really appreciate all the people and families it afflicts, often our own. Until we are informed enough, impatient enough and brave enough to finally and publicly say without embarrassment, "my mother, my father, my sister, my friend, my child, myself," solutions—although visible and achievable—will remain beyond our grasp. That's a choice. It's our move. Together, we could change it. We need to.

EPILOGUE

The last six years of travel and talks have been exhilarating and exhausting. I am grateful for the work I have been privileged to do with students over those years and for the strong and supportive allies who have allowed me the opportunity to do it and who selflessly collaborated in my efforts: Dartmouth Health's CEO Dr. Joanne Conroy, who has been a champion of my work on mental health awareness and fully understands the critical need to create a vibrant mental health system in America; Dr. Barbara Van Dahlen, whose genius in creating the Five Signs inspired me to act; Peter Evers, the former CEO of Riverbend Community Health, and Dr. Bill Gunn, the former director of Behavioral Health at Concord Hospital, who so generously shared their expertise whenever I asked and worked tirelessly to help organize, recruit and launch the awareness campaign in 2016 that we co-chaired; New Hampshire Commissioner of Education Frank Edelblut, who joined me almost 20 times at schools all across New Hampshire to introduce my talk and bolster my plea to students to help change the culture around mental health;

countless friends and supporters, and my incredible assistant Peggy Haskett, whose organizational and collaborative skills made it all possible. My wife and my sons have supported and encouraged my every step during my six-year odyssey. Without them, I wouldn't have found the resolve to even try. I intend to continue to speak and advocate for mental health awareness and meaningful change in mental health access, especially for children and young adults, for as long as the invitations keep coming.

On many of my long rides home these last six years on backroads and interstate highways, I have often tried to connect the disparate dots of my professional life that put me on this path and allowed me to end my career advocating for those suffering from mental illness. But it seems clear to me now. As a trial lawyer, I worked to get justice for clients; as chief justice, I had the constitutional responsibility to administer the justice system; as a law school dean, I was entrusted with training those who would pledge to do justice. As an advocate, now doing the most important work of my life, I want to rectify the injustice done to so many, by so many, for so many generations. I was part of the problem, but no longer. I am impatient for change. Nothing can justify inaction one day longer. Nothing. I need your help, your impatience and your voice.

ACKNOWLEDGMENTS

So many people have made my journey to discovery possible. I can never adequately thank them for allowing and supporting the most important work of my entire professional life, but I will try. First, to all of my colleagues at Dartmouth Health: John Kacavas, whose friendship and constant encouragement made my odyssey move forever forward; Jennifer Gilkie of Communications and Marketing, who saw the possibilities in our campaign, encouraged my efforts at every turn and enlarged my reach; Karen Borgstrom of External Affairs, whose competence and incredible commitment to my work inspired me to try harder; Dr. Will Torrey, for his endless patience and wise counsel whenever I reached out and who always assured me that treatment works; and Creative Services for all their exceptional skills that captured my talks on video to allow my journey to touch thousands of students and adults virtually, especially during Covid-19. Beyond Dartmouth Health, my thanks goes to former Vermont Attorney General TJ Donovan and former New Hampshire Attorney General Gordon MacDonald, who joined me many times at schools to speak to students; former Chief Justice Robert Lynn of New Hampshire, who made time to join me at schools in support of my message; Barrett Christina of the New Hampshire School Boards Association, who opened doors for our campaign and always had time to listen; Dr. Carl Ladd, who reached out to New Hampshire school superintendents to encourage invitations for my school visits; therapist Jeff Levin of the Reconnection Project, who supported and often inspired my resolve for change and greatly educated me about the challenges children are facing; all the members of our steering committee, who gave us wise advice and credibility as the campaign began; Steve Ahnen, who generously rallied the New Hampshire Hospital Association to our cause and provided gravitas for my efforts; New Hampshire Speaker of the House Shawn Jasper and New Hampshire Senate President Chuck Morse, who opened the State House to our launch six years ago and spoke passionately and convincingly about our mission; Tom Raffio of Delta Dental, who gave me countless hours of radio time to talk about the awareness campaign and always lifted my spirits; to my assistant Annette Moore, who diligently kept track of my mileage and expenses and always made me feel like my travel and talks mattered; Lynda Cutrell of 99 Faces, whose brilliant exhibit helped me make the case for change; Karen Jantzen of Riverbend Community Mental Health, whose never-stop, never-quit attitude helped make our launch at the State House so successful; Scott Spradling, whose media experience, savvy and big heart helped spread the word and fill the State House that Monday morning in May; Alex Walker of Catholic Medical Center and Dick Anagnost who gave me free billboard space to display the Five Signs in the critical early months of the campaign; Shannon Disilets in Governor Sununu's office, who helped amplify my message whenever and however she could; Governor Sununu, Senators Jeanne Shaheen and Maggie Hassan, Congressman Chris Pappas and Congresswoman Annie Kuster, who showed up at the State House on day one and generously lent their voices and influence to my efforts; and finally, the countless caring and committed school principals, counselors, teachers and students who helped spread the word about our campaign, embraced my visits and opened my eyes. I am especially grateful to Maura Scully, whose editing skills and wise advice improved my manuscript.

ABOUT THE AUTHOR

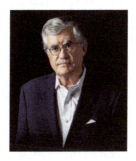

The Hon. John T. Broderick, Jr. was a civil trial lawyer in New Hampshire for 22 years, something he dreamed of becoming since the seventh grade. He graduated from College of the Holy Cross and the University of Virginia School of Law. He served on the New Hampshire Supreme Court for 15 years, seven of those years as its chief justice. After leaving the court, he became dean of the law school at the University of New Hampshire.

Because of his oldest son's unrecognized suffering with mental illness that began when he was 13 years old, and John's mistakes in failing to see it for what it was and deal with it appropriately, his family went on a very public and painful journey in New Hampshire. But they all survived and healed. During the last six years with the unfailing support of Dartmouth Health, for whom he now works, John has traveled almost 100,000 miles in his black Jeep throughout New England to start a new and different conversation on mental health. He has talked to tens of thousands of middle school and high school students in countless gyms and auditoriums about mental health awareness and has spoken to tens of thousands of adults, too. He describes his odyssey as the most important work he has ever done.

In his travels on backroads and highways to speak to audiences of all ages, his eyes have been opened to all the people and families dealing with mental health challenges who are too often struggling to find care. As a result of all the many hugs and confided conversations he has experienced in his travels these last six years, he is fiercely committed to changing the shameful culture and stigma around mental illness that have kept too many people feeling alone, afraid and in the shadows for generations. He is dedicated to doing all he can—especially for children—to advocate for a real mental health system in America. We have never had one.

John currently serves as senior director of External Affairs at Dartmouth Health, serving communities in New Hampshire and Vermont.

Lightning Source UK Ltd.
Milton Keynes UK
UKHW021815281122
412972UK00011B/157